MW01234939

Later

*A Journey of Hope
for When Everyone Survives*

W. E. (Bill) Smith

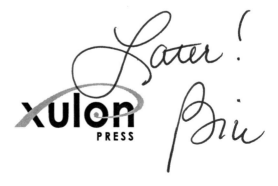

xulon
PRESS

Copyright © 2009 by W. E. (Bill) Smith

Later
A Journey of Hope for When Everyone Survives
by W. E. (Bill) Smith

Printed in the United States of America

ISBN 9781615792689

All rights reserved solely by the author. The author guarantees all contents are original and do not infringe upon the legal rights of any other person or work. No part of this book may be reproduced in any form without the permission of the author. The views expressed in this book are not necessarily those of the publisher.

Unless otherwise noted, all Scripture citations are from The New Revised Standard Version / QuickVerse for Windows Version 3.0h. Copyright © 1992–1994 by Craig Rairdin and Parsons Technology, Inc.

Scripture quotations marked AMP are from THE AMPLIFIED BIBLE: OLD TESTAMENT. Copyright ©1962, 1964 by Zondervan (used by permission); and from THE AMPLIFIED BIBLE: NEW TESTAMENT. Copyright © 1958 by the Lockman Foundation (used by permission).

Scripture quotations marked NIV are from THE HOLY BIBLE: NEW INTERNATIONAL VERSION®. Copyright © 1973, 1978, 1984 by International Bible Society. Used by permission of Zondervan Publishing House.

www.xulonpress.com

Dedications

First, to Claire, the woman who provided Wes with his sweet spirit, a woman who at the age of fourteen was gracious enough to accept a date invitation from a brash fifteen-year-old, and now, more than four decades later, still lights up my days with her smile and her loving Christian spirit. Without her wisdom, love, and support, my life would lack understanding, direction, and purpose.

Second, to our children, Sean, Brittany, and Wes. Their love, sense of humor, and laughter have filled our lives and our hearts with such great times that it makes life worthwhile.

Third, to our many friends, our family, and the church family at Smoke Rise Baptist Church in Stone Mountain, Georgia. Their love and support propped us up in difficult times, and their undying interest in our circumstances and encouragement to send e-mail reports led to the foundation from which this manuscript was developed. The community of faith resides in each of them, and they continue to support us to this day.

Last, but certainly not least, to the doctors and staff at Emory University Hospital in Atlanta. Their wisdom, compassion, love, and understanding made an unpleasant situation bearable. Rarely were they found to lack a kind word, an available ear, or a compassionate heart. Angels can wear scrubs and do at Emory.

Above all, I give praise to God for all our blessings, for the sacrifice of His Son, for His grace and forgiveness, and for His unwavering guidance through the storm.

Contents

1

Triskaidekaphobia

I guess it has to do with blame. When things don't go right, it is human nature to find a scapegoat, something to which you can neatly affix the blame. That's where superstition comes in. According to the *American Heritage Dictionary of the English Language*, superstition is defined as "a belief that some action or circumstance not logically related to a course of events influences its outcome." You know, you'll have seven years of bad luck for breaking a mirror; something bad will happen if a black cat crosses your path in the direction you're headed; bad things will happen if you walk under a ladder, put a hat on the bed or shoes on the table; or, probably the most prodigious, that bad things happen on the thirteenth of the month, especially if it falls on a Friday. That's known as triskaideka-phobia, the fear of the number thirteen.

My dad was extremely superstitious and tris-kaidekaphobic, so I suppose I inherited the phobia. Then I passed it on to my wife. In our defense, there was a pattern in our life revolving around the thir-teenth of the month, most particularly, the thirteenth of February. Let me explain.

At the age of twenty-six, I was married with two children and working in the family business, a new car dealership in Metro Atlanta. On Monday morning, February 13, 1978, at 7:00 AM, as I was preparing to attend a training class sponsored by our franchisor, the telephone rang. My dad was on the other end and said he'd been advised that there was a fire at the dealership. He then asked if I would swing by and check it out on the way to class. I, of course, agreed.

Expecting to find a small three-hundred-dollar electrical fire, I was surprised to find Highway 78 closed off by two fire trucks and a police car two blocks before I got to the dealership. Highway 78 is a main artery running east-west through the city of Atlanta. As I drove around the barricade, I probably thought to myself, "Don't they know there's a fire up here? They can't just close off Highway 78 at this time of the morning."

Upon arriving I found the front of the dealership engulfed in flames as a result of burglary and arson. Seven firefighting units were taking part in extinguishing the fire, and the sky was filled with gray-black smoke. Our records were being shuttled out to the parking lot in huge washtubs, carried by two firemen, one on each side. Once in the lot, the tub was dumped into a heaping pile, and our records were drowned with a water hose to assure no residual embers were active. Local TV and radio stations showed up to record the calamity, but I was in no mood for interviews.

A quarter of a million dollars and 120 days later, we were finally back in business. As one might imagine, this bolstered my dad's fear of the thirteenth and piqued my own curiosity, making me wonder about the validity of his claims.

Four years later, to the day, on February 13, 1982, my dad died. It was a Saturday. He'd been ill and hospitalized for two and a half years prior to his death, so though we were anticipating his death, we still weren't prepared for it. By now, I was

becoming pretty firmly entrenched in the triskaid-
ekaphobic camp. But this story isn't about my dad
(as much as I still love him and miss him) and his
fear of the number thirteen. It is about the circumstances that began on February 13, 2004, twenty-
two years to the day from my dad's death. It was a
Friday. Friday, the thirteenth.

Actually, to fully understand, I need you to go
back to the August following my dad's death. On
August 1, 1982, our third child, Wesley, came into
the world. Born with a pneumothorax (an air bubble
outside the lung between the lung and the ribcage),
Wes remained in ICU for the first few days until
the bubble aspirated. During that time, my wife
Claire wasn't allowed out of bed, and Wes, due to
his condition, was not allowed out of the ICU. I was
allowed to see Wes if I took the proper precautions
of scrubbing up and donning a surgical mask and
gown.

The room in prenatal ICU was painted a light
green, and the lighting was very dim. There were
about eight incubators in the room, and there was
almost a hallowed reverence to the manner with
which the nurses attended to this space and the
lives it protected. Other than an occasional blip or

bleep of a monitor, the only sound was that of a radio on a wall shelf, quietly playing rock music. I would sit for as long as they would let me, holding Wes, rocking him in the rocking chair there in ICU, listening to the rock music channel on the radio. Despite my attempts to quietly sing to him during those few short visits, we bonded.

Irrespective of his difficulty at beginning life, Wes became a pretty healthy kid. Other than having a slight touch of asthma and experiencing the scrapes, bruises, cuts, and colds that most kids get, he had always been in good health and was an especially loving and giving individual with a gentle spirit. In grammar school he would willingly give his lunch money away to another child who had none. He would let his friends play with his toys until they broke them, and then Wes would take the blame, never wanting to show his friends in a bad light. He was a team player.

Team sports were a challenge for Wes because he was small. But he rose to that challenge and succeeded in basketball and soccer. As a fancy-dribbling point guard, he'd sink three-pointers from about anywhere on the basketball court. As either a right- or left-wing forward and equally adept with either foot, Wes could kick a soccer ball past the goalkeeper into the corner of the net so fast that the keeper never saw it. Then Wes, with his blond hair streaming behind him and his arms lifted to the sky, would run full blast back to his high school teammates and leap into the group, forcing them to catch him. After exchanging hugs and pats, they'd do it all over again.

Wes also excelled at individual sports. In our family and among his friends, Wes's skills at ping-pong, bowling, and golf were formidable. Few things gave him more pleasure than "pasting" someone at a game of ping-pong, unless it was pasting someone at the bowling lanes. His best round of golf was a score of thirty-seven on nine holes with a par of thirty-six. One over is pretty exceptional. I often encouraged him to take lessons, but he repeatedly refused. "Dad, I just don't have the time. I just want to enjoy what I do."

I got the same response from Wes when I tried to get him to take piano lessons. Self-taught, Wes composed some beautiful pieces. Our piano is in our living room that's centrally located in our home. The room has a twenty-two-foot-high ceiling and a catwalk connects one side of the upstairs to the

other, so as Wes would sit for hours, playing varia-
tions of the same tune over and over again until he
had it just right, his melodic presence was audible
throughout the house.

Unable to read music or write it, those composi-
tions were never transcribed. He just didn't have the
time.

After high school, Wes had some difficulty
finding his center and his area of interest. I think he
had intended to follow in his dad's and granddad's
footsteps in the automobile business, but I had since
sold the dealerships, so Wes's love for cars was
manifested in the pride he took in modifying and
showing his own car. He worked odd jobs, attended
a local community college, and spent every spare
minute changing and improving his car. First, it
was an Acura Type R that he entered in the NOPI
Nationals, the quintessential car show for cars
of this nature. He won. The following year, Wes
entered his new car, a Honda S2000, in the NOPI
Nationals and won again. This was his passion.

Having finished most of his core-curriculum
material at the local community college, Wes just
didn't know what he wanted to do. A friend of mine
suggested Savannah College of Art and Design

(SCAD). When I made the suggestion to Wes, he lit up. Wes had taken art in high school and was quite talented. To my surprise he took the initiative to get the application, fill it out, produce his portfolio for judging, and (along with Brandon, his friend and future roommate) was accepted to start in the fall of 2003. His focus was architecture.

Savannah, Georgia's oldest city (having been founded in February of 1733 as a haven for England's working poor and a buffer between the English settlements in South Carolina and the Spanish presence in Florida), is steeped in historic architecture. During the Civil War, General Sherman burned down Atlanta and everything else in his path on his March to the Sea, but when he arrived in Savannah, he was so struck by her beauty that he refused to burn it and offered it to President Lincoln as a Christmas present. Because of the general's compassion for the city—its beauty and its history— Savannah is filled to this day with elegant, historic architecture, ornate ironwork, fountains, courtyards, and green space within the city. The college was founded in 1978 by a few folks from Atlanta's art college. They designed a curriculum that provided an excellent arts education and inspired students to exercise their creativity in many ways. Lacking a centralized campus, SCAD began purchasing buildings in downtown Savannah to house various classrooms, one building here, another there, until today, Savannah College of Art and Design is the largest single property owner in all of downtown Savannah. As a result, dormitory space in Savannah was limited and sometimes not convenient to wherever class might have been scheduled in the city, so Wes and Brandon rented an apartment in Savannah on one of the islands that dot the Georgia coastline. At least that was the story Wes and Brandon gave the parents, and we fell for it. I would suspect it had more to do with the cool swimming pool, the club house, and the close proximity to the beach.

They moved down in June, in advance of the school year, to find part-time employment and get the "lay of the land." They got the lay of the land all right. They had a blast. They'd go to the beach in the morning, work a few hours in the afternoon, and party all night. Then classes started in the fall and caused them to make only some minor alterations to their already hectic schedule. SCAD was great for Wes. He loved the school, loved the city, loved the people, loved learning, and had found his niche.

By now, we were in the late fall, early winter of 2003. When Wes came home or we talked with him on the phone, he seemed to have some minor malady akin to a cold or the sniffles. Over-the-counter remedies worked for a while.

In the second week of February 2004, Wes called his mom and admitted to having missed a major test at school because he had just felt too sick to attend. His professor had hung on policy and refused to allow Wes to make up the exam without a doctor's excuse. Wes wanted to come home to see the family doctor and get the excuse he needed to return to class.

Having been exposed to enough triskaideka-phobic thinking to have developed her own fear of the date, Claire begged Wes to drive home on Thursday, the twelfth of February, so that he wouldn't be on the road on Friday the thirteenth. He agreed, and she made the doctor's appointment for Friday with our family doctor who had been seeing me for about forty years. He was my dad's doctor and was now seeing the third generation of Smiths.

Surprisingly, I don't think when I awoke and got ready that morning that I thought much about it being Friday the thirteenth. I had scheduled a meeting with some gentlemen regarding the formation of a new bank, and Claire and Wes were going to the doctor to get Wes a note and maybe some medication because he looked a little puny.

Claire, however, had no intention of going with Wes to the doctor. When she asked him when he was leaving, he asked, "Aren't you going with me?" Her reply must have stunned Wes because she said, "Wes, you're twenty-one years old. You can go to the doctor by yourself." Wes then said he really wanted her to go with him, so she did.

In this day and age, cell phones are a blessing and a curse. It's wonderful to have their availability, but annoying if they interrupt what you're trying to do. During my rather protracted meeting that stretched into and beyond lunch, my cell phone never rang, despite my discourteous habit of leaving it on and activated while attending meetings. Upon exiting the restaurant, I looked at my phone and the screen indicated two missed calls. There had been no ring, no indication whatsoever that a call had been received. As I sat in the car and stared at my phone, I couldn't get over how odd the feeling was that my phone had apparently malfunctioned and failed to alert me of an incoming call or even a message. It had most likely been Claire with the results of Wes's appointment. Though I didn't have reason to be fearful over his appointment, for some reason I felt eerily uneasy.

Attempting to hold that feeling at bay, I listened to my first message. It was Claire. "Smitty, call me right away." That was all it said. Short and cryptic is uncharacteristic for Claire. Then the second call: "Smitty, call me. We're at the emergency room at Emory. Wes has leukemia."

2

How We Heard

Stunned, dazed, confused, I raised my eyes to the sky and asked the question that anyone would normally ask after receiving such horrendous news, "Why?" I knew the question was rhetorical, but somehow I had hoped for an audible answer. There was none.

I called Claire's phone and got voice mail. Undaunted, I tried again. Same response. Third time, same thing.

I sat in the parking lot in my car and buried my head in my hands and said to myself, "Okay, Bill, keep calm. Think! What should I do now? What do I know?" I realized that I knew that Wes was in the emergency room at Emory University Hospital in Atlanta. I had to get there as fast as I could.

Fortunately, law enforcement on Interstate 85 South took a holiday on that Friday the thirteenth. Interstate 85 is a main thoroughfare through Atlanta. Going southbound, I significantly exceeded the speed limit in two counties on my way to Emory. Somehow, maneuvering in and out of traffic, I managed to carry on a rather incomplete conversation with myself on the way. "What *is* leukemia?" "How did Wes get it?" "Why him?" "Why us?" "Why me?"

Periodically recognizing that my conversational partner wasn't responding, I attempted to reach Claire by cell phone, each time receiving voice mail. Either her phone was turned off, or she was in a location where the signal wouldn't reach. Finally, I decided to try Wes's phone. I rationalized that he had a different cell phone service that might reach when Claire's wouldn't. Connection was made, and I got directions from Claire on how to find them in the hospital. Not wanting to waste time, I valeted my car and ran inside.

Once inside those huge emergency room doors, Wes's room was the first one on the left. It was

a hospital room about twelve feet by eight feet.
Within was any type of monitoring equipment
necessary for emergency patients. The room's small
dimensions left little room for visitors or family to
sit and wonder what was about to happen. There I
found Wes—scared, pale, eyes puffy from crying—
lying on a gurney. There, too, I found Claire—
scared, pale, eyes puffy from crying—sitting on the
edge of the gurney holding tightly to Wes's hand.
At that moment I had too few arms and too few lips.
I didn't know which one to hold and kiss first. I
started with Wes.

As nurses and doctors entered and left Wes's
room—sometimes with testing equipment, sometimes with needles—I intently watched Wes's reaction to what was going on around him and to him.
They poked, prodded, and stuck him. He never
flinched. He was going to fight. He, as we, knew
little about leukemia, its cause, its treatment, or its
rate of cure, but Wes was determined that if he had to
be the dog in this fight, there was going to be lots of
fight in the dog. He started fighting leukemia in that
very room on that very afternoon. He would not quit.

As tests went on, I was able to periodically ask
Claire what had happened at the doctor's office. She

explained that after looking at Wes, they ordered a blood test. The nurse tech drew the blood and sent it back to the lab. They waited. After a while, the physician's assistant (PA) reentered the room and said she had to take another sample. She assured them that such an incident was fairly routine, as it was not uncommon for samples to become contaminated. After a while, the doctor and his PA reentered the examining room.

Dr. Walz became my doctor when I was fourteen years old and trying out for high school football. He'd been my dad's doctor and had been treating him for years prior to my dad's death. Dr. Walz was a stocky man with a grayish-red beard and thinning hair. He was in his late sixties and spoke with a slight New York accent as a result of his medical training at a New York university. He had a gruff voice from years of smoking cigarettes and then cigars.

"Claire," said the doctor, "I believe he's got something bad."

Now, Claire and I had discussed the possibilities of Wes's illness. He had complained about some back pain, so we assumed that he either had pneumonia or the strain of spinal meningitis that seems to proliferate on college campuses. We were wrong.

"I think Wes has leukemia."

Claire had probably been less stunned when the same doctor had diagnosed a lump in her own breast some seven years before. It is one thing to fight your own demon and quite another to think that your child is faced with one. Shocked and speechless, Wes and Claire looked at each other.

The doctor then asked, "Who was your oncologist at Emory and is that where you want to go?"

Claire confirmed those intentions and gave the oncologist's name to the doctor so he could begin the referral process. Claire and Wes were then left in the room alone. There, they broke down together and wept.

In between the sobs and the tears, they comforted each other. Claire rationalized and told Wes that this leukemia is an *L* word not a *C* (cancer) word. "We can get through this, Wes," Claire assured. "I've been through this type of thing before, and I'll show you how. If I can do it, you can do it. You'll see."

After a while, the doctor returned to tell Claire that the emergency room at Emory was waiting for Wes and that they should head over there now.

Once in the car, Claire looked at Wes and asked "Do you know how to get to Emory?" He didn't.

Back in they went to the doctor's office. The nurse needed only to explain the first major road, and it came back to Claire how to go. Back in the car they went.

Once at the emergency room, having finally made contact with me, Claire had called Wes's older brother, Sean, and tried to reach his sister, Brittany, on her cell phone. Britt is a hairdresser at a salon in the Buckhead section of Atlanta. As a professional rule, Britt does not answer her cell phone when it rings, if she's with a client. When Claire called, Brittany was with a client, and on this particular day Britt and her client Shirley were discussing cancer. Shirley's husband was currently going through some advanced stages of cancer treatment as was my brother Claude. Britt told Shirley about Claire's battle with breast cancer as the incessant cell phone continued to ring. Finally, to her relief, it stopped.

A few minutes later, as Britt and Shirley resumed their conversation, one of Britt's coworkers interrupted. Initially perturbed by the interruption, Britt turned to see Bernice looking very pale and worried as she handed Britt the salon phone. Claire, not wanting to unduly alarm Britt in a public setting, summoned her to Emory without offering a reason. Britt would not be satisfied with that lack of information.

Was it Papa (Claire's father who had recently suffered a stroke)? "No," Claire replied.

"Is it Dad?"

"No."

"Oh, my God, is it you?"

"No, it's not me," Claire replied.

"Is it Sean?"

"No, Britt, it's Wes. They think he has leukemia."

As each question had been asked and answered, Britt slowly slid down the salon wall until she was sitting on the floor, sobbing, oblivious to the stares of other patrons who wondered what was going on. Upon explaining the call to her client and apologizing that she had to leave her in the middle of her appointment, Shirley said, "Come on, Britt. I'll take you to Emory." And so she did.

Upon Britt's timid entry into the emergency room, she found Claire and me. As difficult as it was to remain strong, we encouraged her to do so for Wes's sake. She straightened her back, sniffed back her tears, and turned to find Wes standing in the doorway, wearing jeans and a sweater and looking not much different than the last time she'd seen him. "How can he be sick?" she thought.

Wes, sensing the gravity of the moment for us all and especially for Britt, looked at her, smiled, and said in a calm and loving voice, "There she is," and reached out to hug her.

About 9:00 PM Wes was admitted into the hospital into a room on the sixth floor in E-wing. By that time Sean had arranged to pick up my eighty-eight-year-old mother and bring her to the hospital. Claire's mom and dad were contacted, as were a couple of close friends. News traveled fast, however, and by 10:00 PM, the halls were filled with neighbors, friends, church members, our pastor, and relatives.

6E, as the name suggests, is on the sixth floor E-wing and is cordoned off from the elevator by double doors. On the wall is a sign that forbids entrants to bring flowers, fresh fruit, or small children. It is a triangular structure with about eight rooms per side and a nurse's station, reception area, staff lockers, refreshment area, and supply closet

in the middle. Patients are rarely seen in the halls
unless they have been instructed by their doctors to
walk. Walking was encouraged to build strength.
Upon our arrival, a woman approached Claire and
said, "Welcome to your home away from home."
We weren't looking for another home, and Claire
thought, "There's no way that this is going to be my
home away from home!"

Eventually, we were able to meet for a short
time with the oncologist. His remarks were rather
cryptic, but his spirit was warm. He calmly and
compassionately advised us that Wes had been
ill for a couple of months. It was very fortunate
that our primary care physician had diagnosed the
leukemia and sent Wes to Emory. Had the leukemia
been allowed to continue over the weekend (due
to its aggressive nature, its exponential effect of
immature white-cell replication, and with Wes's
white blood count already at 140,000), Wes would
have been blind or dead by Monday. Chemotherapy
would start immediately. We'd talk more over the
next few days about his treatment regimen.

At 1:00 AM on Saturday, February 14,
Valentine's Day, Wes began receiving his first round
of chemo. We observed him for a couple of hours

to be certain that he didn't exhibit any adverse reactions, and then, once he was asleep, Claire and I left to go home for a few hours of much-needed sleep.

3

Getting a Grip

We slept about three hours, rose, showered, dressed, and prepared to go back to the hospital. Prior to leaving the house, I sent out the first of what turned out to be a series of e-mails regarding Wes and the state of the Smith family. The first one was sent to one of our Sunday-school class leaders. This lady does a wonderful job disseminating information to other class members and acts as a gatekeeper for news, prayer concerns, and praises.

Little did we know that first Saturday morning how badly we would tax her abilities, her patience, and her commitment to her seemingly thankless, unpaid job of Internet queen.

The message was pretty direct and to the point that morning and explained that "we don't know what we don't know." We knew so little about leukemia, what we didn't know seemed infinite. We lacked so much knowledge, we didn't know what to expect from Wes, the doctors, or the disease.

Armed with this knowledge vacuum, Claire and I started out that morning for our second of about three hundred trips from Duluth to Decatur, from home to Emory. We didn't know what to expect or what we'd find once we arrived. We were tired, scared, and confused but dedicated to saving our son from the unknown. We knew little about the disease, less about the chemotherapy, and even less about how either or both would affect Wes.

Most mornings, that trip was a blur, forgotten upon arrival and generally accomplished by sheer reflex. Looking back, making that trip as often as we did with less attention to driving than should have been given, it's obvious that our cars seemed to be guided by remote control as the direction, speed, and lack of accidents delivered us to the parking deck at Emory without incident each day. Emory University's roots were established in 1836 by the grant of a state charter to the Methodist

Church conference. Oddly enough, its forebearer hospital was Wesley Memorial Hospital and was chartered in 1904 with financial support from the founder of the Coca-Cola Company, Asa Candler. The hospital was moved to its current location in 1922 on the campus of the university on Clifton Road, six miles northeast of downtown Atlanta, and has been expanded many times over the years. It began establishing itself as a first-rate teaching hospital for nurses and doctors. The name of Wesley Memorial Hospital was changed in 1932 to Emory University Hospital. The main building, the Whitehead Memorial Building, which now acts as the face of the hospital by housing the lobby and the administrative offices as well as the emergency entrance, is a five-story limestone-veneered building constructed in the federalist style with a huge center pediment. It is screened from the road by huge oak trees that overhang Clifton Road and give an imposing reality to the massiveness of the complex.

We parked in the seven-story concrete parking deck located behind the medical office buildings and clinics across the street from the hospital. Those buildings are connected to the hospital by a glass-walled, enclosed bridge that spans Clifton Road. That morning we traversed that bridge for the first of many times. On that bridge we would encounter medical staff dictating test results into a cell phone or tape recorder, visitors remarking about the patient they just saw, family members crying over a patient's condition or rejoicing as they prepared to take him or her home. We would, in time, learn to identify some of those faces and, as we would find out, identify with the emotions as well.

The chemo began attacking the leukemia cells quickly. Wes's color was better and his eyes appeared stronger than they had. Dr. Winton poked his head in the door and made this warm yet cryptic remark that gave us hope: "You're doing beautifully. We've got them on the run."

We took heart in Dr. Winton's words and Wes's general appearance. Wes had started to feel better. Despite being hooked up to an IV pole hung with numerous bags of constantly dripping IV fluids with lines running into his arms, he started to show a bit of a sense of humor. He was constantly tethered to this pole with rollers; wherever Wes went, so went the pole. Wes decided that every companion should have a name, so he named his IV pole "Gilbert."

Anytime he would rise, he would address his pal, "Come on, Gilbert, I've gotta pee . . ."

In less than twenty-four hours, Wes had already won the hearts of most of the nursing staff and most of the physicians with his sense of humor and sweet spirit. They'd obviously not had anyone name an IV pole before and had probably never seen one adorned with pink-and-white handlebar streamers and a pink bulb horn that Sean had picked up at a toy store and affixed to "Gilbert" in an attempt to lighten Wes's spirits. Gilbert took on his own persona.

Sean, ten years Wes's senior, is about an inch shorter than Wes with reddish-blond spiked hair. He is trim, athletic, and muscular. Trendy in his dress, he and Wes had become quite close over the last few years playing recreational soccer on various teams around the Atlanta area. Together, they were a force to be reckoned with. Anticipating each others' moves when they played forward positions in a game, Sean and Wes would pass without looking and each would intercept the ball, dump back to the other, and seemingly score at will.

It was evident that Sean was having difficulty with Wes's illness. He'd always dealt with things

much differently than other people. Not necessarily efficiently, but differently. In his earlier years,
having been known to overreact to situations, he
learned how to detach himself, thereby making it an
easier task to regulate his feelings. He had decided
long ago that not exhibiting emotions would keep
him from spiraling out of control. It didn't mean he
didn't have feelings; he just adamantly refused to
express them. If he could rationalize the minutest
detail of a situation, he could cope. Wes's disease
was no different.

Sean, as did the rest of us, knew little of this
disease called leukemia. But he was certain, as we
all were, that this had been caught early, and in
2004, few people actually died from leukemia. After
all, his mom had beaten breast cancer seven years
earlier. Fortunately, we live in the United States
with some of the most advanced medical technolo-
gies available in the world. Two of Sean's friends
had been diagnosed with leukemia years earlier and
both were in full remission. When Sean came by
the hospital, characteristic of his detached self, he
usually remained fairly quiet. Then, when you'd
least expect it, he would pepper the conversation
with an occasional sarcastic joke. Wes loved him

deeply and seemed to appreciate Sean's sense of humor.

Brittany scarcely left his side. She is six years older, but she and Wes became the best of friends. They were party buddies. They would meet up a couple of times a week at some night spot in the Buckhead area of Atlanta, and there they shared friends and laughs. They both had a sense of humor and were classified as two of the funniest people we'd ever met. Each could have qualified as a stand-up comedian. They could usually find humor in any situation. Wes's illness, however, was different. The leukemia hit Brittany hard. She wanted to will him well. Whatever he wanted, she'd do. She tried to help him eat the hospital food and, when that tactic failed, she ran out to get him a burger or fries from outside the hospital. She was dedicated to her brother.

Due to our lack of sleep the night before, the exhaustion generated by that loss, and the stress created by the situation, Claire and I had secretly hoped for a few minutes to close our eyes during the day and take a nap. We needed the rest. What we got was a steady stream of visitors bearing gifts and food that kept us busy every moment of that first day. Relatives and friends from the church or the neighborhood came steadily throughout the day, often bringing forbidden gifts like flowers or fresh fruit. All asked the same question. "Why?" We, too, yearned for the answer to that question. Nonetheless, telling and retelling the story and explaining how little we knew became tedious. We realized that these people cared enough to ask about Wes and our well-being. They meant well, and we just needed to persevere. We could sleep later, much later.

Wes, too, was feeling the effects of the stress of the situation. He blew off a little steam at one of the nurse techs in a somewhat sarcastic manner. When this little sprite of a woman came in to take Wes's vitals, she retrieved the blood-pressure cuff from the wall, strung the coil cord across the bed, and due to the placement of his IV pole, hooked the cord over the side rail to secure it. Once the cuff was affixed to his arm and inflated, she was intently listening and watching for a reading when, without warning, the coil cord—stretched to its limit—slipped off the guard rail and snapped straight, slapping Wes in the head. "Hey, woman," Wes said, "I just find out I have leukemia, and then you slap me in the head with the equipment! What are you trying to do? Kill me?"

Not knowing Wes or his sense of humor, the remark obviously hurt her feelings. She left the room, returned a little while later having been crying, and apologized to Wes. Wes felt bad for having hurt her and apologized to her as well. The hug that followed started a fast friendship of love and respect between the two of them that would serve them both well in the journey ahead.

The chemo treatments needed to be spaced out by twenty-four hours. Typically, that would mean that Wes's second treatment wouldn't begin until Sunday at 1:00 AM, so we were in for a long day and night. In an effort to attempt to get Wes on some sort of normal schedule, the doctors reasoned that they could cheat the treatments by one hour each night. Over the course of the treatment, this would slowly move his end time down to a reasonable hour.

We stayed that second night until about 2:00 AM, watching Wes sleep as he received his chemo. With no adverse reaction evident, we slipped out again and went home for a few more hours of much-needed rest.

Upon arising Sunday morning, I called the nurses' station on 6E and asked to speak with Wes's nurse. She assured me that Wes had experienced an uneventful night and that was great news. "Uneventful" meant that he had had no adverse reactions, no allergic reactions, no problems at all. No news was indeed good news.

Sunday morning was fairly quiet at the hospital. I suppose it was due to the fact that our church friends were at church. But following church hours and into the evening, visitors came in streams. Sometime that second day during a lull in visitation, Dr. Winton entered Wes's room and asked to address us all regarding Wes's illness. Even our lack of sleep could not prevent us from being "all ears" for his words.

Now, Dr. Winton is a stately, silver-haired bespectacled oncologist in his mid to late sixties who is never seen without his white lab coat. He is a man of few words, but those words he offers are calm and kind. He has the demeanor and delivery that can tell you bad news and have you accept it. Fortunately, on this day, the news wasn't bad. The bad news had been a couple of days before when Wes had been diagnosed with leukemia.

Dr. Winton sat down next to Wes's bed and addressed Wes as he allowed us to intentionally eavesdrop. This is basically what he said.

Wes had Acute Myelogenous Leukemia (AML). To understand the disease, one must first understand how the blood system works. Typically, stem cells replicate to make more cells. Initially, these new cells are undifferentiated. As they begin to mature, they do a couple of things. One, they differentiate themselves from the other cells by deciding whether they will be white cells that fight infections, red blood cells that carry oxygen, cells that "take out the trash," as Dr. Winton described it, or various other types of effective cell types. Second, they establish a life span for themselves, determining how long they will live and perform their function before they die and make room for other cells of their type. If an individual has been exposed to a nuclear blast or has come in repeated contact with a chemical used in oil refineries (benzene) or simply possesses a mutant genome, one of those stem cells could mutate into a clonal or leukemia "blast" cell. That's right. Just one cell starts this whole mess. One becomes two, two become four, four become eight, eight become sixteen, and so on. These cells replicate without differentiating what they'll be. They never establish the apoptosis process by which they determine their life span, and they, therefore, continue to divide and replicate without maturing. As they do this, they start taking up space normally inhabited by good cells. They continue to crowd out the good guys and fill up the system with unproductive, unhelpful cells. Without efforts to stop them, the patient's organs no longer receive the blood or help they would receive from healthy blood cells and, as a result, those organs begin to fail. Due to the small capillaries in the eyes, when white counts rise uncontrollably with blast cells, these small blood vessels get clogged up first and the result can be temporary or permanent blindness. This was about where Wes was when he was admitted. A typical white count is 8,000 to 10,000, 14,000 if you're fighting an infection. Wes's white count was 140,000 when he was admitted to Emory. Above 200,000 can be lethal.

Wes began the induction phase of his chemotherapy with a dose of cytarabine. He would receive six infusions of cytarabine over six days. He would begin the first of three doses of daunorubicin tonight. Due to its color and characteristics, daunorubicin is known as one of the "red devil" drugs. The side effects are not pleasing, but it is part of the conventional treatment for AML patients.

Upon completion of this round of chemotherapy and within twelve days from the onset of treatment, Wes's white count would begin to drop precipitously as cells began to die. The target would be the blast cells. In reality, good cells would die too. The result would leave Wes susceptible to any type of infection or bug with which he made contact. He would have to be quarantined during the week to ten days while the white count rebuilt with what was hoped would be healthy cells. Doctors would watch his progress closely during this time. The best-case scenario would have Wes in the hospital for twenty-one days, out for ten, back in for six, out for twenty-one, back for six, and so on until all five rounds of chemotherapy were completed. The first two would include the daunorubicin, the last three only the cytarabine. There was a 20 percent chance that the induction phase would have to be repeated and that would add to the daunorubicin infusions.

Wes was unhappy that he would be hospitalized for a minimum of twenty-one days. He'd hoped to be released by Saturday. But there were some bits of good news in Dr. Winton's remarks. Wes was not in the high-risk group. AML usually strikes adults in their mid to late sixties who already have medical conditions that make treatment and recovery more difficult, like high blood pressure, heart disease, diabetes, kidney problems, etc. Given that fact and Wes's otherwise good health, his likelihood of going into remission after treatment was 80 percent. Remission would be monitored by a series of bone marrow biopsies conducted on specific days following chemo treatments to determine if blast cells were resident in his bone marrow. Even if they were not evident in the bloodstream, if they were in the bone marrow, eventually, they'd be in the blood.

We didn't talk much about Dr. Winton's comments once he left. Honestly, we didn't have much of an opportunity. The parade of visitors and well-wishers continued.

We hung around until Wes started to receive his chemo and then slipped out for home. The trip northbound on I-85 was considerably quicker in the wee hours of the morning than in the heat of the day.

We followed our regimen fairly religiously over the next week or so, rising each morning to make the trip to the hospital, sitting with Wes, attending to visitors, and waiting with bated breath for some word from his oncologist. Those words were few and short, but sweet.

"We're encouraged by what we see . . ."

"You're doing great!"

"I wish I could move the calendar for you . . ."

"I'm glad you don't feel bad enough that you want to be here . . ."

"Keep it up."

"Walk some . . ."

Whatever morsels of good words or news we could get, we sucked them in and savored them for all they were worth. We all needed those encouraging words.

The other encouragement we received was from the white count we had quoted to us each day. If you recall, the white count on the day of Wes's admission was 140,000 and going up. Now, the count was trending down. As we approached the last day of this round of chemotherapy, Wes's counts were down to 2,200. Needless to say, the chemo was kicking his butt pretty good, so he slept most of the day.

Following that last round, his counts dropped another step to 800. His doctor came in with the exclamation, "You're doing great!" Wes's eyesight had improved, and after a short nap in the afternoon, he was fairly alert and seemed to be regaining some of his steam. We could tell this by his explanation of how he had "fired" his assigned nurse who was on until 11:00 PM because his late nurse was a "hottie."

Saturday was not a good day. Wes felt lousy in general, didn't eat much, and slept quite a bit. On Sunday he recovered somewhat and had a ravenous appetite for anything other than hospital food. We brought food in, Sean brought food in, and Britt brought food in. So did some of his friends. He had continued to lose weight over the week he'd been hospitalized, so it did us good to see him eat, regardless of what it was.

Early into the diagnosis and hospitalization, Dr. Winton had suggested that Wes might need a bone marrow transplant or the more common stem cell transplant. Little did we know that in 1979, Emory was the first hospital in Georgia to perform a bone marrow transplant. Pioneering medical procedures was not uncommon to Emory; they had been the first in the state to transplant corneas, lungs, kidneys, a pancreas, liver, and heart, as well as changing cardiology forever with Dr. Andreas Gruentzig's inventive heart procedure of angioplasty. Still, our ignorance of Emory's history was only surpassed by our ignorance of how and what bone marrow transplants entailed.

To accomplish the bone marrow transplant, a suitable donor would need to be found. Preferably, this donor's DNA would match ten of ten markers for which they test. Of course, Claire and I eagerly volunteered but were jointly devastated when it was explained how unlikely it was that either of us would be a suitable donor. "But we're his parents," we persisted. Here's how it was explained.

"Wes is a product of the two of you. Each of you has different DNA from the other. Wes's DNA is a combination of both DNAs you bring to the union. At best, either of you would be only a 50 percent match. It is more likely that one of Wes's siblings would be a closer match as they, too, are products of the both of you."

On the second Monday following Wes's admission, Sean and Britt were both tested to see if they were suitable donors. It would be weeks before the results came back.

4

Fevers, Drugs, and Varsity Burgers

W hen Claire underwent treatment for breast cancer in 1997, we recognized that cancer patients and those who love them live their lives in installments. The installments are created by the two extremes of fear and hope. When tests are due or results are awaited, fear consumes you. Once the results are received and they are good, you're able to relax with the hope that bad news has been held at bay until the next test. The test schedule dictates the frequency of the installments.

That being said, our emotions ran up and down the fear meter during the course of Wes's first two weeks. Alternating between fear and elation was new territory for me. I was uncomfortable with it. I had always been somewhat of a control freak. I had been forced into managerial roles in my early twenties due to my dad's illness. I had the responsibility of 120 employees and their families. I had been forced to learn that, if something was wrong, I couldn't rely on anyone to take responsibility for the issue and fix it other than myself. If I had a difficult situation, I found a way to fix it or change the situation. I was unable to do either under these circumstances. I was at the beck and call of this disease called leukemia. Everything that took place did so at the schedule dictated by the illness. Little did I know how much more difficult this personal, internal conflict would become.

Wes tried to adjust to life in the hospital. In particular, Wes initially found an aspect of his stay somewhat uncomfortable. That happened to be Thursdays. Emory University Hospital is a teaching hospital that's trained thousands of medical professionals over the years. Thursday was the day when the medical professors made rounds with the medical students. They would enter a patient's room, circle around the bed, and stare as if they were looking at a monkey in a cage. Then they would take turns poking and prodding and asking questions: some profound, others stupid. They would then exit and move in a herd down the hall, first pausing in the hallway to review the chart and prepare themselves for the genus of monkey in the next room. Wes endured the procedure but would occasionally (on days when he felt less well) ask me to see if I could ask them to skip his room. They always accommodated when asked.

The treatment regimen dictated that a bone marrow biopsy be done on Friday to see if any of the leukemic blast cells remained resident in the bone marrow. The twice daily blood tests indicated that there were no blasts in the blood and that was a good thing. However, since blood is manufactured in the marrow, if leukemic blast cells are found there, it's only a matter of time before they will be found in the blood.

A bone marrow biopsy involves taking a large hypodermic needle and inserting it into the pelvic bone down to the marrow and extracting marrow fluid. It is a painful procedure for which patients are given localized anesthetic, usually Demerol, and a drug called Versed. Now as we understand it, Versed isn't as much an anesthetic as it is an amnesic drug that alters the mind so that, while under its influence, you don't remember the pain. It was discovered early on that Wes's body seemed somewhat resistant to both and, therefore, required much more than the average patient to generate the desired effect. They obviously got this one right as Wes had no complaints upon his return.

We got what we believed to be good news that afternoon when one of Wes's doctors came in and said that initial indications showed no blasts in the sample. That being said, they were still going to conduct more tests over the weekend and provide final results on Monday. The tests that they were going to do involved fluorocytometry. Fluorocytometry involves injecting the sample with certain agents that bind with the proteins that are unique to and surround leukemic cells. Microscopically viewing the sample will then cause any remaining resident leukemia blasts to fluoresce or glow.

I didn't want to wait until Monday. Once again, what I wanted didn't matter.

That weekend, Wes developed a mysterious fever of unknown origin (FUO). Due to his depressed white count, he had been on some rather generic antibiotics to ward off any potential problems. The hospital decided to bring out the "big guns" and chose to put him on an intravenous drip of Vancomycin (Vanco). Typically, the infusion time is one hour. Within fifteen minutes of his being hooked up to the Vanco, Wes's face and head turned beet red, and he started clawing at himself, itching uncontrollably. When we alerted the nurse on duty assigned to Wes, she strolled in, took one look, and casually said, "Oh, he has red man's syndrome."

Now, this was the first time as parents that we'd experienced our son having a side effect to any of the medications. We thought a more urgent reaction would have been in order from the nurse. Little did we know, she was responding properly but calmly by retrieving Benadryl to administer by IV. She did and, despite the Benadryl taking quite some time to calm him, Wes eventually drifted off to sleep, exhausted and drugged.

Monday afternoon, the doctor came back in to apprise us of the results of the bone marrow biopsy. Apparently, the sample showed some curious markers, but all of the professionals who viewed the results remained confident that the results were not leukemic involvement. Trusting them at their professional word, we felt some sense of relief that they were going to begin Wes on his Neupogen, or growth-factor shots, in an attempt to prepare him for release. These growth-factor shots, administered by subcutaneous injection (a short needle inserted in the fleshy tissue just below the skin's surface), would stimulate the system to make new blood cells and bring his counts back up to normal levels. Once his white count returned to normal, he could go home. He was all about that.

It would be an understatement to say that Wes was never a fan of hospital food. Being the cagey soul he was, he learned early on that there was some benefit to be derived from being sick. He had all of us, his mom and dad, sister, brother, and most of his friends at his beck and call to bring him food from the outside at any time. Once he discovered that there was an alternative to hospital food, I don't think he ever ate it again.

Now the Varsity, for those of you not from Atlanta, is a hot dog diner started in the fifties by a Georgia Tech University dropout and established at North Avenue and Interstate 85 near the campus of the college. At one time, the comedian Nipsy Russell was reportedly a carhop at the Varsity.

Known mostly for their hotdogs, chili, and onion rings, the Varsity serves delicious food, even though it might be called a little, how shall I say it, "greasy." On a good day, a healthy person can experience gastronomical surprises by eating too much Varsity food.

Wes was never a big guy, weight wise. As I'd mentioned earlier, he was always the smallest on the basketball and soccer teams. However, sometime in his junior year of high school, Wes went through a growth spurt and added about a foot onto his height. The weight didn't come with it. He was always lean, rarely above 127 pounds. Now, battling the leukemia and dealing with the side effects of chemo, he was really thin, six feet two inches tall and 107 pounds, so we encouraged him to eat however and whenever we could, Varsity or otherwise. His appetite was an important building block in his recovery.

Therefore, we were quite delighted to enter his room one afternoon to find Wes sitting up in bed, eating chili dogs and onion rings, grinning like a Cheshire cat the whole time for having conned his friend into making the Varsity run and delivery. Seeing this, with his attitude improving, the doctors started making noises about letting him go home. He was thrilled by those prospects, but to be truthful with his counts so extremely low, we were ambivalent about our role as caregivers to an adult who had been cooped up for three weeks in a hospital, particularly someone who would be susceptible to any bacteria or fungus he might encounter. Again, control—or the lack thereof—became a big issue.

5

Have a Nice Day

At 9:30 PM on March 4, we arrived home with our precious cargo. Wes was extremely proud of his dismissal. Early on, the doctors had said the best-case scenario would be twenty-one days in the hospital and then out. Wes was dismissed on the twentieth day. He had been personally and secretly working for that dismissal date because it represented a better scenario than best case. He was released one day earlier than what the doctors originally thought, and he was convinced that by being a better patient and beating those odds, he could beat leukemia too. We shared and rejoiced with him in his accomplishment and enthusiasm.

Needless to say, we were relieved to have this respite from hospital visitation and the constant vigil it required. Freedom felt like a new condition, so we decided to embrace it cautiously. You might even call our venture mundane. Claire needed a haircut.

Now, taking a trip to the stylist may seem routine and boring to some, but to us on that first day, it was worthy of celebration. We were elated to have the opportunity to go together (just the two of us) to visit Brittany at her salon in Buckhead.

As part of our celebration, we decided to drive my little red sports car that had been held hostage in the garage for the last three weeks due to Wes's circumstances. Listening to its powerful little engine purr and feeling the acceleration as we, once again, headed south on I-85 just added to the thrill of the freedom.

Freedom does have its limits.

Within a half mile of our exit, we were cruising southward at what I thought was the speed of traffic, thinking out loud about nothing and everything, listening to the radio, and trying to embrace this shackleless existence. I looked up and discovered that my rearview mirror was filled with flashing lights. I was being stopped by the Georgia State Patrol.

Now, I'm normally a fairly affable guy, and when given the opportunity to discuss a situation, I can be fairly persuasive, but today, given the totality of the circumstances, I wasn't feeling all that affable.

I nervously waited for the officer to approach my car. I rationalized that, if I could talk to him, I could tell him my story and convince him that a warning would suffice. I just hoped he'd be receptive and compassionate.

He wasn't. He wasn't a *he* at all. He was a *she*. And she had an attitude and was a woman of few words.

"License and registration? Court date and the phone number are on the front of the ticket. Have a nice day."

She turned on the heel of her freshly polished boot, returned to the ubiquitous blue-and-gray cruiser, and left. The fog she created by her exhaust couldn't have been as thick as the fog of disbelief that had permeated our car by her visit. Claire and I looked at each other completely stunned. Eighty-two in a fifty-five.

What else could happen to us? Keep reading. The future was equally unbelievable.

Wes enjoyed his time at home. He had friends visit him. He put the top down on his car and went to visit them. He played the piano. He generally pushed the envelope of what the doctors said he should do. If he went to eat with friends, we encouraged him to eat on the patio, stay away from crowds, and wash his hands often.

During this time, his hair fell out. Having been warned of the occurrence and in anticipation of it, he'd had his sister give him a buzz cut. Once the buzz started falling out, he just shaved his head. Surprisingly, it looked natural on Wes. Tall and lean, Wes wore his baldness like a badge of courage. He would push his pair of Oakley sunglasses on top of his head, hold his head high, and strut wherever he went. Other than a somewhat paler complexion than normal, no one had any indication that Wes wasn't the picture of health.

Wes was also a comedian. There was nothing about leukemia that was going to stop that. You need a mental picture of this. There was a character for the Six Flags theme parks who was a skinny old man with a bald head and these huge glasses. Prior to his illness, Wes would imitate this character's mannerisms perfectly. After his treatments and hair loss, I found a pair of huge dark-rimmed sunglasses at a drug store in Emory Village, took them back to Wes's hospital room, popped the dark lenses out, and handed them to Wes. You'd have thought I'd given him a pony. He loved them and would entertain visitors, doctors, and nurses alike.

One day, while we were stopped at a traffic light on a trip back from the clinic, Wes said, "Watch this." He bent over and disappeared from view of the driver in the car to our right. While bent over double, he put on the glasses and rose back into view, looking right at the other driver and smiled just like the old man from the Six Flags commercials. I thought the driver was going to have an accident he was laughing so hard. All the way home, Wes messed with other drivers. Unfortunately, leukemia continued to mess with Wes.

During his time at home, trips were made back to Emory clinic on a regular basis to check his blood and administer blood transfusions or platelets as needed. During this time, his PICC line malfunctioned.

When Wes was first admitted, he had to endure constant needle sticks for the administration of his chemotherapy, antibiotics, medications, and general fluids. Time and time again, the nurses would come in and insert a needle into a fresh or not-so-fresh vein to accomplish the task at hand. Wes never complained. He'd make a face and flinch a little, but he never said anything about it. It was the doctor who suggested that a PICC (peripherally inserted central catheter) line with multiple leads be installed to facilitate the administration of the drugs without constantly having to stick Wes each time. Wes was taken down to radiology and had a PICC line installed. It did make things easier to some degree.

PICC lines must be flushed each day to prevent any bacterial buildup or blood clots from forming. That was a learning experience for Claire as she was pressed into the service of seeing that was done. Likewise, Wes had to be given those subcutaneous shots to build up his white blood count. Claire learned to administer those as well. Though Wes learned to give himself the subcutaneous shots, he preferred that his mother give those to him. Sterile dressings surrounding the PICC had to be changed, and it was general gymnastics for Wes to take a shower without getting the dressings wet. Homecare was not a piece of cake, and Claire, more so than I, found herself learning to do things that she never thought she could. But a parent's love is without boundaries. A parent will do whatever it takes to save his or her child.

The time at home was good. We developed a routine of scheduled dosing of medications and trips to the clinic for blood and/or platelets. Claire managed Wes's medications and the administration of injections and infusions. I don't know how she kept it all straight. Occasionally, she wouldn't, and Wes, pretending to be asleep, would rouse just long enough to say, "It's two, Mom, not one." Wes owned his disease and, when necessary, took complete responsibility for his treatment. Despite his willingness to do that, we kept close tabs on Wes while still allowing him to have the freedom that he needed to actually live and recognize some benefit for not being in the hospital.

Wes was scheduled to go back in the hospital the next Thursday. Mentally, he and we were better prepared because we thought we knew what to expect. He was to be in for six days. He was to take the same chemotherapy he had taken before, and he figured he had some idea of how he would tolerate it. He did not have to eat hospital food if he didn't want it, and the routine that had served him so well on his first round would likely be there for this one. The time was drawing close.

During this time at home, Wes, always a sensitive child, had become fond of sitting in the grand room of our home, looking westward out the large palladium window and soaking in the kaleidoscope provided by the sunsets each afternoon. Often, he would summon Claire or me to sit with him to watch as the hues of blue, orange, purple, and pink changed by the minute and the shards of light broke between clouds as the sun sank lower and lower behind the tree line until it disappeared beyond the horizon. It was the majesty of it all that seemed to mesmerize Wes. It was as if God was putting on a show for Wes, and he didn't want to miss a single act.

6

Round Two

Surprisingly, when it came time for Wes to go back in the hospital for his second round of chemo, he accepted his fate and decided that he would make the best of it. He called the nurses on 6E and, as if it were a five-star hotel, requested a room with a view. He got it. Embarrassed at the time by his presumption, I am to this day amazed at how accommodating the staff at Emory was to Wes and how forgiving they were for his making the most outlandish requests. Wes had a way of asking that didn't seem as if he assumed some entitlement to have his request granted but a sense of knowing that certain things could be done if requested. As a result, Emory made what could have been a difficult stay much brighter.

And so it went. Thursday we reentered Emory for the second round. We had to be at Emory at 7:45 AM for Wes to have a new PICC line installed. After the procedure was accomplished without complication, we sat around until about 11:00 AM while they got his room ready. Once there, we settled into our hospital routine.

Wes did get a room with a view. It was a corner room with a large window that—unlike his first room that overlooked a narrow courtyard with the view of another building—faced west and looked out over the Emory University soccer fields. During the day, he could watch the students practice, and in the evening he could watch the sun set. Given his prognosis, those sunsets seemed to take on a new meaning for Wes. After checking the clock, he'd say, "Dad, open the blinds." And then he'd soak in every nuance of the event.

During the day, Wes would watch TV or sleep, Claire would read books or magazines, and I would work crossword puzzles. It was important for us to just be there for Wes. As a result, the crossword puzzles were a release for me. I'd sometimes work a dozen a day. Occasionally, visitors would come by. Claire and I would slip out to the cafeteria, the student food court, or a restaurant at Emory Village for lunch.

Emory Village is located at the end of North Decatur Road, a main thoroughfare in Dekalb County. It's a little hamlet with a pizzeria, a pub, a sandwich shop, a drug store, and a few retail shops that support the college students who are housed nearby.

Upon our return to the room, we would stay until about 7:00 PM, and then we would leave, find a location close by the hospital for dinner where we could decompress with a glass of wine and a meal, and then drive home to Duluth where I would answer e-mails and Claire would answer voice mails. Then, after another glass of wine and a cigar for me, we would collapse into bed only to arise and do it again the next day.

It probably sounds dull, but it was a system that offered me some of the control I felt I'd lost to the disease. It was important for us to take care of ourselves. We were, after all, the caregivers. Who cares for the caregivers, if not themselves?

Fortunately, in the evenings about 7:30, Britt or Sean would bring Wes dinner from outside and stay with him until later in the evening. Brittany commonly stayed until the wee hours of the morning, if not all night. During these stays, Wes, depending upon his strength, wanted to walk the halls. The doctors encouraged this, and Wes obviously felt that maintaining his strength was a catalyst to recovery. Britt would walk with Wes sometimes while he was tethered to his IV pole. He would always speak to other patients, doctors, and staff and was affable in a precocious kind of way. Often, when meeting a lab tech or nurse approaching from the other direction, he would hold onto his IV pole and pretend to play "chicken" with them, testing them to see who would be the first to yield. Then he would just laugh and chide them for not showing more nerve.

Britt tells of countless times when Wes would walk by the nurses' station and catch someone's eye behind the counter. He would then deftly execute the old vaudevillian routine where he dropped slightly lower with each step he took until he disappeared below the edge of the counter as if he had descended steps. "Going down!" he would say to Britt's embarrassment and to the nurses' laughter.

67

Similarly, either his brother or one of Wes's friends showed consistent love and support by coming early in the morning with breakfast and staying until our arrival about 10:00 AM. Wes never wanted to be without people around and with this schedule and cast of supporters, he rarely was.

One of Wes's friends, an Estonian by the name of Raivo, was especially dedicated. More mornings than we can count, we found Raivo sitting in Wes's room when we arrived, having spent the night with Wes and gone out and brought him breakfast so that Wes would be spared the injustice of hospital food.

The first infusion of this second round of treatment was somewhat uneventful, so uneventful that the following day we were able to take him to the student food court for lunch where he was able to enjoy the sunshine and the real world.

The second infusion was a different story, and though we were able to once again get him out, food was not at the top of his wish list as the nausea began to take its toll. We did manage to get a little food in him prior to the third night's treatment. But he experienced some pain while receiving this one. The following day was another day of simply enduring the side effects.

Earlier it had been mentioned that due to Wes's age and otherwise good health, a remission rate could be expected with probability as high as 80 percent. If the remission came about quickly and periodic bone marrow biopsies showed no blast cell activity, there was a 40 percent chance that the leukemia would not return. That, of course, meant that there was a 60 percent chance that it would. The only real cure for leukemia was for the patient to undergo a bone marrow or stem cell transplant. Let me try to explain in nonclinical terms what I believe I know about each.

When it was first reasoned that the blood cells start in the bone marrow and that blood diseases might be cured by replacing faulty bone marrow, clinicians attempted to match up donors for the afflicted patients and bone marrow was extracted from the donor by use of a long needle and injected into the recipient in the same manner. It was a painful process for both.

Subsequently, it was realized that blood cells develop from the stem cells of bone marrow and that the blood stream has stem cells resident in it. By utilization of the same machine that separates red cells from white cells from platelets, researchers had found that blood could be extracted, spun at a different velocity, and the resultant remainder would be stem cells. Once the stem cells were extracted, the remainder of the blood could be reinfused into the donor. The stem cells could then be infused just like a blood transfusion into the recipient.

Sounds simple, but for the recipient it's not. Here's why.

The afflicted recipient needs to be in remission for at least three to four weeks prior to being admitted for transplant. Once admitted, he or she receives a high-dose chemotherapy treatment that causes those treatments previously received to pale in significance. Heretofore, the chemo drugs would allow regeneration of the patient's own blood supply. The high-dose chemo administered prior to transplantation is so strong, it kills all of the patient's blood-making capabilities. Once destroyed, those blood-making capabilities will not come back. This is by design to prevent recurrence of the blast cells.

A calculated period of time must elapse to allow the chemo time to do its work. During this period, as it goes about its business killing good cells and bad, it begins to kill out the bone marrow. This can and often does cause significant bone pain in the patient. Consequently, the patient feels really lousy.

Then, once the stem cells are infused, they start to work attempting to become acclimated to the new surroundings. They go about making blood, but it's the blood type of the donor, not the patient. As a result, the new blood begins to recognize organs foreign to its type and begins creating white blood cells to fight off these organs. If not controlled, the blood will reject the patient. This is commonly referred to as graft versus host (GVH) disease and can be fatal. Doctors have a delicate balancing act in the administration of immunosuppressive drugs to prevent this rejection. If the procedure is successful, the blood and body will typically acclimate to each other in about ninety days, and the patient will start feeling better. In the meantime, the cure is often thought worse than the disease.

The patient must continue to be monitored closely for at least a year, sometimes much longer. The act of stripping away the immunosuppressive drugs is a tedious maneuver that can bring on life-threatening complications. It is always the patient's desire, as it is the doctor's, for the patient to live without drugs. However, impatience with respect to discontinuation of these drugs can cost the patient his or her life any time up to and including two years or more posttransplant.

Suffice it to say, transplant is a risky proposition. Though it is the only known cure for leukemia, once in remission, the transplant procedure doesn't contain significantly better odds of survival. Nonetheless, it is the only known cure.

Not knowing what turn Wes's recovery would take, the doctors had suggested that he might be a candidate for a stem cell transplant. We accepted that possibility.

The criteria tested for suitability of a donor are numerous. As mentioned previously, it has to do with DNA typing, and the doctors prefer a perfect match. However, a related sibling donor may be acceptable even if a few markers don't match. It was hopeful that Brittany or Sean would be the perfect match for Wes. Neither was.

As a result, a search was done for an anonymous donor from the International Registry. The search was at our expense and fairly costly. Insurance would pay for harvesting the cells and the resulting transplant but not for finding the donor. Matching DNA is like finding a needle in a haystack, and DNA typing is time consuming and expensive. Irrespective of the costs involved, we asked the hospital to pursue finding a donor for Wes.

During the second installment of chemotherapy at the hospital, the term started out fairly mild. As the treatment progressed, however, the situation became a little more problematic. The results of the last bone marrow biopsy indicated more problems.

Dr. Winton came in that afternoon to tell us that residual blast cells were found in Wes's test sample. This meant that the induction phase would need to be repeated, so Wes would receive six rounds rather than five. Though this was not the news we had hoped to get, Dr. Winton went on to say that due to Wes's extremely high white count upon first diagnosis, it would have been considered a rarity if he had gone into complete remission after only one round. The doctors did not seem to be concerned about the findings.

They also found a small blood clot in the vein housing Wes's PICC line. Upon receiving his last infusion of this round, Wes would have his PICC line removed, and he would be sent home with a blood thinner in addition to the myriad of other medications. It was just something else to add to our list of worries. Something else we couldn't control.

7

Not-So-Good Friday

Wes came home after his second round of chemo. The results of chemotherapy are cumulative, so it was apparent that Wes didn't feel quite as good after the second round as he had after the first. Similarly, some of the antibiotics had side effects that weakened his appetite and caused him to be pretty grumpy. We had been warned and were prepared, but it was still rather disconcerting when all our energy was expended toward making him well and those efforts seemed unappreciated.

Easter was upon us, and Claire and I had always prepared lunch for the family and had an Easter egg hunt for the kids of our extended family at our house. Last year, as all the children were getting older, we had changed the method of the hunt by hiding only one egg per child. Each egg had one child's name written on it and inside was a ten-dollar bill. If they found someone else's egg, they couldn't divulge the discovery. They were instructed to simply place it back where they found it and wait for the right party to discover it. The difficulty of the hiding places was directly proportionate to their ages. The older they were, the more ingenious the hiding place. Some were inside birdhouses. Some were in rain gutter downspouts. Wes's was inside the tailpipe of his car. Everyone found Wes's egg except for Wes. He had been pretty frustrated, but it was funny. Remembering last year's hunt made us eager to replicate it this year. However, Wes's clinic schedule had him returning to the clinic on Easter Sunday. Those visits generally took a minimum of five hours, so Easter plans were scrapped.

On the evening of Good Friday, Wes mentioned a slight pain in the right side of his back, just above the kidney. We all hoped that the pain would subside with the ongoing antibiotics he was taking. It persisted until Easter Sunday when it became more painful, and his temperature shot up to 104 degrees while at the clinic. The nurses immediately called the doctors, and Wes was readmitted to Emory that day.

The next morning, they scheduled Wes for a bronchoscopy. Upon completion of the test, their suspicions were confirmed. Wes had pneumonia. The "big gun" antibiotics were called out. They were very strong, and Wes seemed to react negatively to one. That reaction was manifested in his temperature going up to and even higher than 106 degrees. When Wes's symptoms were not improved by the administration of these drugs and after an inconclusive CT scan of his lungs, the doctors reasoned that the infection must be fungal. Fungal infections are extremely hard to treat and eliminate. There are basically only three known effective antifungal agents available for use with patients. A needle biopsy of Wes's right lung was conducted to attempt to identify the type of fungus causing the pneumonia. Prior to receiving the results of the biopsy, the doctors guessed which fungus was responsible, changed his drug regimen to include this antifungal, and were successful in generating immediate results. Irrespective of their success, Wes's spirits were dampened by his once again being in the hospital on a holiday and the fact that Easter was much different than previously planned.

Coincident with our attempts to save Wes from this insidious disease, my sister-in-law was fighting a similar battle in an attempt to save my brother Claude, four and a half years my senior, who had battled and apparently beaten Hodgkin's disease only to have been diagnosed with esophageal cancer a little more than a year ago. It's quite possible that the esophageal cancer was a result of the acid reflux created by the chemotherapy administered to fight the lymphoma. Life is sometimes not fair. The prospects for anyone with esophageal cancer are dim, but more so for someone who has not fully recovered from the treatment necessary to fight off another form of cancer. He was experiencing mysterious fevers and seizures, and the prognosis was not good.

This was something else over which I was unable to exercise my otherwise characteristic control. The next day was no different.

The following day, Wes was scheduled for a needle biopsy of his right lung. He was, therefore, NPO (nothing by mouth) after midnight the night before. Someone lost his orders, and they didn't come to get him until 2:30 PM. Needless to say, Wes was hungry and irritable. We kept trying to explain that there was a possibility that someone in the ER might have needed to have a procedure done to save his or her life and that Wes's procedure would, in that case, be of a lesser priority. That seemed to help until they brought him back in about two hours without having done the procedure. Apparently, having had nothing to eat or drink for about fifteen hours had dehydrated Wes to a point that his blood pressure dropped to a level unsafe to perform the biopsy.

He managed to cajole the attendants into getting him two turkey sandwiches before he got back to the room, but he was still angry. We tried to commiserate with him, but he'd have none of it.

As luck, or bad luck, would have it, an appointment with the bone marrow transplant director was scheduled for that day. She called and asked if he was still up for the discussion, and he relented, unwillingly, to meet with her.

Dr. Langston, Amy, as she prefers to be called, is in her midforties with brownish-blond hair and small wire-rimmed glasses. Prior to coming to Emory, she had been trained at one of the preeminent bone marrow transplant centers in the country, the Fred Hutchinson Cancer Institute in Seattle, Washington. She is rarely seen without her white lab coat and arrived that day adorned with various pins on her lapels. One of the pins was pink, about the size of a half dollar, and was emblazoned with the words "Cancer Sucks!" Wes hated that pin. He probably hated it for two reasons. One, he assumed that she'd never had cancer so she couldn't possibly know the degree to which cancer did, in fact, suck. Second, her patients had already determined that cancer sucked so by wearing the pin, she was just adding insult to injury. Her presentation put Wes in an even fouler mood.

Still, after all we had been through, we tried to listen to what she had to say. Little of it was encouraging. That wasn't Dr. Langston's fault. It was just the nature of the discussion. I think all of us, Wes included, simply catalogued the information and filed it away hoping it would never be needed. The discussion was cryptic. When the doctor was finished, we went back to Wes's room and didn't discuss it further.

Then, as if Wes's illness was insufficient to overwhelm us, on April 23, 2004, my brother passed away. My mother and his family were with him when he died. Once again, I suffered from this lack of control. I felt it important to be with my brother during his last few days or hours, but didn't feel that I could leave my son.

So just when I thought that life was as unfair a mistress as could be found, she took another turn. The antifungal medications began to work their magic, and the doctors released Wes to go home.

8

Miss Charlotte

Some weeks earlier, during our clinic visits, we kept seeing these two folks about our age coming and going, always with smiles on their faces. She was receiving treatments for a blood-borne cancer, and he was her caregiver. He came by and introduced himself as Charles Williams from Chauncey, Georgia (a small town, southeast of Macon), and his wife Charlotte. Charlotte was always the epitome of a gentle-spirited Southern belle. Charles was always full of nonsense and making people laugh with his antics, jokes, or impersonations. It was obvious that they were genuine, loving people, and we all fell in love with

Charles and Charlotte, Wes included. Little did we know how close a parallel our lives would develop.

Flashback

Shortly after our first meeting, I received an e-mail from Charles indicating that they had not received the news for which they were hoping. Charlotte's counts were wildly fluctuating. The e-mail was to let us know that until Charlotte's blood could be stabilized, little could be done at Emory to prepare her for the stem cell transplant. For that reason, they were sent home to monitor her blood work and schedule a return once it was stabilized.

Charles always signed off with "Expect the best!" Always upbeat, Charles really did expect the best, felt like he got the best when he married Charlotte, but was having a hard time reconciling Charlotte's cancer with the best outcome. He, too, must have felt out of control. But Charles rarely let that feeling show.

As we got to know Miss Charlotte and Charles better, we found that Charlotte had been an administrator with the school system "back home" and that Charles followed his dad into the new car business down in Eastman, Georgia, at about the same time that I had joined my dad in ours. Both having been Ford dealers and both of us the same age, surely our paths had crossed in that previous business life. Charles left the car business to spend some time in the banking business. Ironically, my other interest and part-time career is in organizing and building community banks. Needless to say, Charles and I had much to talk about.

Charles loved Charlotte with every ounce of his being. It was evident anytime he was around her. And why not? Who wouldn't? Her countenance was so gentle and sweet. Her makeup and hair were always perfect. Her ensemble always complimentary to her coloration and style. Her beautiful looks belied her condition. She was preparing for a BMT, bone marrow transplant. Lucky for her, one of her sisters was a perfect match.

Charlotte had a tumor resident in her upper right shoulder that radiation had been unsuccessful in eliminating. Upon irradiation, it would shrink and then return to its previous size. The doctor's hope was that, once transplanted, the internal struggle for position created by the transplant would attack the tumor and eradicate it. First, they had to get her blood stabilized. Charles and Charlotte continued to weave in and out of Wes's story.

On Sunday, April 25th, I received the following news from Charles. "Charlotte's dad passed away Friday, April 23rd. We are home for the funeral, and it is a very difficult time indeed."

This was unbelievably surreal. My response to Charles was, "What a coincidence. My brother passed away the same day. It wasn't sudden. It was expected, but it was still a shock. We go to Greenville, South Carolina, tomorrow for the funeral."

On Monday, the 26th of April, Claire and I traveled to Greenville to attend my brother's funeral. Wes was at home with his friends calling and looking in on him.

My eighty-eight-year-old mother was the picture of grace and strength under pressure. Only about four feet eight inches tall, she towered over most at the funeral, maintaining decorum and composure when others of younger age and firmity seemed less equipped. When it was revealed that in my brother's last moments, my mother stood over him and quoted the 23rd Psalm, word for word from memory in a voice stronger than her eighty-eight years would allow, it was apparent to me that she was one to look up to despite my more-than-one-foot height advantage.

The service was emotional, as one would expect, and was made even more so by the appearance of some of our friends from Atlanta who made the trip under poor weather conditions just to support us. Throughout our journey with Wes, the one thing that brought me to tears more quickly than anything else was the compassion of strangers. Well, maybe not total strangers, but folks that you knew, but you didn't know they cared as much as they did. Those revelations caught me gasping for air. I'd often heard the phrase "taking your breath away," but it wasn't until Wes's illness that I actually experienced that phenomenon.

They say that the measure of a man can be judged by the size of his funeral. Well, though my brother Claude was a man small in stature (five feet one inch), he was seven feet tall in the hearts of many, judging by the attendance at the memorial service that afternoon. It was a wonderful service, appropriate to honor a wonderful son, brother, husband, father, grandfather, friend, artist, and humanitarian. He would be missed by all.

My mother, Carol (his wife), his daughter, son, and grandson were the picture of grace and strength during the ceremony. Drawing on their faith and the friendships of many, they managed to celebrate Claude's life as we all said good-bye. I admired them all for their poise and courage.

Wes and I spent the following day in the clinic and the result was a report that his counts were good and his recovery was to the point that the doctor wanted to reinstate him to Emory on Monday to begin his next round of chemo. He was then given permission by his doctors to go to Savannah to visit his friends and check on his apartment over the next few days. By now he was acutely aware of his treatment regimen, and we, as parents, had mixed emotions about his trip. We knew it would do him a lot of good to see his friends and he'd be healthier to receive his next round as a result.

Often, when our lives are in turmoil, we tend to wear blinders regarding other events, however traumatic they may be. Occasionally, one slips through the defense screen and slaps you back into reality. One such event occurred that following weekend.

We live in a large neighborhood, so it's not unusual that we don't know all our neighbors.

One of those neighborhood families experienced a tragedy when their nine-year-old daughter died in a horseback riding accident. Here was a family that, through no fault of their own, had a child snatched from their home and life. Can life be so fragile? So brief? How devastating must it be to suddenly lose a child? The recognition that the candle can be snuffed out with no warning gave us pause over our efforts to cure Wes. What a blessing it was that we could attempt to provide care that might render him well. They had no such opportunity.

9

The Other Miss Charlotte

Wes enjoyed his trip to Savannah to visit his friends, furniture, and stuff, but by returning a day early, he spoke silent volumes about his condition. Not due back until Sunday, Wes indicated he was ready to get on with his next round of treatment with his Saturday return. Much to our surprise, even that didn't go according to plan.

After making an attempt to admit Wes to the hospital, we discovered that the CT scan performed prior to his leaving the hospital the last time didn't really show the type of improvement Wes's doctors had hoped. In turn they thought that the antifungal should have some more time to work, so we were scheduled to visit the clinic each day for administration of the antifungal, and on Wednesday a port (big brother to a PICC line) was to be installed so that Wes could be readmitted on Friday for further chemotherapy treatments.

Friends continued to show their genuine concern with inquires and comments that offered hope as evidenced by the exchange following my last e-mail announcing the postponement of Wes's treatment.

"So, this is a good thing?"

"We think. I guess. Who knows? Maybe. We hope. Thanks."

"Is Wes still planning to check in for a treatment tomorrow?"

"Ask us tomorrow. Just kidding. We think maybe, if nothing changes when he goes for infusion today, and the moon's in the right phase, and the doctor's in a good mood, and they synchronize the traffic lights on Clifton Road, he's supposed to go in tomorrow morning or afternoon or before midnight."

Each day we rose to face a new day within which we could exercise little if any control. We surrendered our son to Emory. We awaited instructions at the end of each day for the next. Then we set our cap on accomplishing just that—nothing more, nothing less, just that. It may seem like a valiant thing for us to do to exercise such restraint. In actuality, we were so stressed, we couldn't process any more than what the next day would bring. The Bible promises strength for the day and reminds us that the past is gone and that tomorrow is yet to come, so we tried desperately to trust God's Word to provide for us by daily installments. I must admit some difficulty in this aspect of my belief. I desperately needed more control.

Bless his heart. Wes so much wanted to celebrate a holiday, any holiday, out of the hospital. Valentine's Day, he was in the hospital. Easter Sunday, he was in the hospital. Mother's Day, he was in the hospital. He was so looking forward to Memorial Day.

Unfortunately, as with the other holidays, Wes spent Memorial Day in the hospital for observation and antibiotics, having run a fever Sunday night. He returned home Tuesday afternoon and was back in the clinic for transfusions on Thursday and Friday. His counts were recovering, and we anticipated getting a date for returning for the next round of chemo when we saw the doctor on Monday. Still no word on whether a transplant was being advised, considered, or scheduled.

It would seem that the rash of seemingly unending bad news would cause us and most especially Wes to question God. With so few ups and so many downs, it would seem that our blessing trough had run dry. Quite the contrary, God continued to bless us in unimaginable ways by placing in our path certain individuals who acted as angels. It happened too often to have been simply rationalized as coincidence because those people came unpredictably and unavoidably into our lives. Many times, their wings were hidden by their scrubs. Such was the case at Emory. In both the clinic and the hospital, angels, with wings obstructed, wrapped their arms and their hearts around us so tightly that we were enveloped by their love each day.

One such angel was a lady by the name, oddly enough, of Charlotte Williams. Not the Charlotte Williams I introduced earlier, but a friend to our family for more than thirty years. Thirty years ago, Charlotte, a recently divorced mother of two young girls, realized it was necessary to seek employment to provide for her daughters. A registered nurse who had taken time off to bear and raise her daughters,

Charlotte lived across the street from us and sought employment with a new division of Emory hospital. Successful in her quest, Charlotte began her new job as an infusion nurse in the newly formed cancer center at Emory University Hospital, working with oncologists Drs. Elliot Winton and Tom Hefner. That first morning, lacking a sitter for her girls, she asked Claire to watch them. So as Charlotte had embarked on her new career, Claire had watched her two daughters.

Charlotte was a dedicated employee and extraordinary caregiver, excelling in her position. When Claire was diagnosed with breast cancer in 1997, Emory seemed the logical place for her treatment. There, Charlotte administered most of Claire's chemotherapy with an uncommon degree of compassion and care. Now, some seven years later, Claire had recovered from her surgery, reconstruction, and treatment, and I was indebted to Charlotte for her love and professionalism. The fact that Claire was healed was due, in large part, to Charlotte's dedication to her job and her undying friendship.

Now, with Wes in a struggle for his health, we called on her again, and she rose to the occasion with an all-too-often rare degree of love for our son, as if he were her own. As if her own dedication were not enough, Charlotte garnered the compassion and love of all the nurses in the infusion center to tend to Wes's every need in such a fashion that we felt they were family. Almost to the extent of feeling guilty, we were accorded every accommodation to make our visits trouble free. Everything we needed to do was streamlined to a point of embarrassment when compared to other patients. We soon realized that we could go through the back door of the infusion center, and Wes's chair, the second one on the right in pod J, would be awaiting him with a warm blanket and hard Scandinavian-designed wood-and-chrome caretaker chairs available for Claire and me. Someone would be waiting to take blood from Wes and get his labs processed, and the pharmacist would occasionally come by to check on Wes and us. As we became more accustomed to the process, we realized that we were not alone in our conveniences. The infusion center demonstrated a degree of compassion and love to all their patients that made them feel special and managed to ease the discomfort that the diseases seemed to create.

As time went on and the frequency of our visits increased, our love for the nurses in the infusion center grew to a proportion that we recognized that any day we arrived for treatment Marie, Judy, Karen, Dana, Lucy, Angela, Carmen, Barbara, Juliet, Rhonda, Claudia, Charlotte, and countless others could be depended upon to show Wes special care, as if he were their own. All came by to speak to Wes each day and to check on his comfort and ours. A warm blanket, a cold drink, and anything else he could desire were available at his request. What a comfort that provided to us, his parents.

Likewise, the hospital staff on 6E and 7E, the leukemia floor and transplant floor, showed us special treatment. There was the cute blond Clemson graduate Wes thought was a "hottie"; the seasoned nurse with answers to most of our questions; the efficient nurse who had once worked for our family chiropractor; the nurse tech who looked at Wes as her own child or grandchild; the nurse who had served for several years in the military and was one of Wes's most-beloved caretakers; the brunette nurse Wes repeatedly proposed to; and others provided a level of compassion and loving care that made us feel confident and comfortable with his care in our absence. Wes could be a handful when he was "in hospital," but they rose to the challenges he consistently created and dealt with his illness and needs in a professional and loving manner.

Emory utilizes physician's assistants (PAs) in a most effective manner. All were wonderful and talented. To fail to mention Marian, Michael, Somie, and others would be remiss on our part, but one, in particular, stole Wes's heart and ours. Jessica, Dr. Winton's beautiful, brunette PA (in her early thirties and with a sweet spirit) not only tended to Wes's every malady and need, but to ours as well. It is unimaginable what our journey would have been like without her wise counsel, experience, and loving demeanor. Whenever times were the most difficult for Wes and us, she was there to soothe our fears with her sweet words and smiling face. To this day, we value her knowledge and friendship.

As an aside, it should be duly noted that the angels employed by Emory, though trying desperately to hide their gossamer wings, were unsuccessful in hiding their loving kindnesses from those they encountered. God is in that place and in the hearts of those people they employ.

10

Something Smells Bad

Chemo treatments in hospital became somewhat routine. Despite an occasional low-
grade fever, Wes tolerated the chemotherapy pretty
well. Because of this, I asked if Wes could sleep
at home each night and come to the clinic to have
his chemo administered. Those treatments would
take about four hours each day. He could eat and
sleep at home and try to live an otherwise normal
life. My request had to be studied at length by the
doctors. It seemed that such a protocol change
had never been requested by anyone, and since
it was out of the ordinary, it was easier to say no
than yes. Undaunted, I persevered, and after some
consternation, the doctors relented and agreed to

that protocol for his next round. Wes went to have his labs checked at the clinic and when the results came back to the doctor's satisfaction, he was once again released for a week and given clearance to go to Savannah. Wasting no time, he and a friend left directly from the clinic and drove to Savannah.

To Wes the magnetism of Savannah must have been freedom and a change of place and pace to forget about the cancer that coursed through his veins. He still had medications that had to be taken each day. While he was away, those were solely his responsibility. I tried not to think about the things I couldn't control when he was out of my care and custody. Other than an occasional pill, shot, or flushing of his PICC lines, those days in Savannah could be filled with that very day and those very friends doing those very things that made Wes the most happy. He could be Wes, and his disease could remain anonymous. For Wes it must have been like turning the clock back to a time before February 13th.

Once again, with Wes released from the hospital and a reprieve at hand for a week, Claire and I experienced that strange feeling of freedom. But this time, with Wes not only being out of the hospital but being out of town as well, that sense of freedom was even more pronounced.

Claire and I decided to take a day trip. The city of Dahlonega and the outlet malls are about an hour north of our home, if you take the back roads.

It was a warmer day than it had been, so once again we broke out the recently neglected little red convertible. The top came down, and we took off. We were both experiencing a certain sense of release—listening to the radio, feeling the breeze, laughing and smiling—when we felt rain.

I'd always thought that it took clouds to make rain, but there wasn't a cloud in the sky. Still, liquid continued to hit the windshield.

Highway 53 is a winding two-lane road that goes east-west from Gainesville to Dawsonville. There are few, if any, places to pass or pull over. We were in a slow procession of cars and trucks that seemed to be going slower and slower. And what was worse, there was an odor in the air that we tried repeatedly to identify and explain. We rationalized that, since we were near or crossing Lake Lanier, there must have been some sort of industrial waste or sewage spill. It would pass as we distanced ourselves from the lake.

With no means of escape from this unwilling but seemingly interminable parade, eventually, we saw a miracle happen in front of us. A fork in the road, heading off to the left. About eight cars directly in front of us peeled off and headed for other destinations.

Finally able to drive above thirty-five miles per hour, we sped up to close the gap to the next-closest vehicle that had traveled over the hill and out of immediate sight. Soon, gap closed, it started raining harder. I turned on the wipers. The windshield became a blur, but that blur provided enough clarity to identify the wetness that had been hitting our car.

Directly in front of us were two eighteen-wheel manure trucks. We had been following them for about eight miles. Properly covered with tarps, the manure, apparently fresh and steaming, caused condensation against the cool air blowing across the tarp and the resultant liquid had been blowing off and behind them for miles.

Not only had the spray found our windshield but our hair and sunglasses. The smell had become so offensive, Claire had pulled her sweater sleeves far past her hands and used the excess to cover her nose and mouth like a mask.

Just as we thought we were going to be forced to close the westbound lanes of Highway 53 in an effort to save ourselves by stopping to put the top up, miraculously, the trucks turned off and clear sailing lay ahead.

We downshifted and accelerated to distance ourselves from the odor as quickly as possible. Still, it seemed omnipresent.

We stopped at the first service station we saw, and I cleaned the windshield three times.

Despite being miles away from the trucks, the smell lingered. It was apparently on our clothes and in our hair. Once we were walking the streets of downtown Dahlonega, it seemed so obvious to us. We feared passersby would give us a strange look and turn up their noses, but none did.

Quite simply, we stank.

That day's journey paralleled another journey, the journey we had been traveling with Wes. It stank too.

With no control over the situation, unable to go left or right, stop or back up, we plodded along hoping for a reprieve. We hoped that the leukemia truck would, as those manure trucks did that day,

leave our path and leave behind only the topical
residue of its visitation.

As we showered that night, we could only hope
that the day would come when we could wash away
the effects our trip through leukemia had already
left on Wes and us. That was our prayer.

Wes once again had gone to Savannah, his new
home, to see his friends and visit his stuff. One
place he loved was the Soda Pop Shop. It's located
in a little storefront about two blocks from the
administration building of SCAD on Bull Street
in downtown Savannah. There are a couple of
café tables outside on the sidewalk and only room
for about four tables on the inside. The counter
stretches across the entire width of the store. It's
been run by two partners for years and is a favorite
with SCAD students as it became for Wes. He
ordered the same thing every time he went: a chili
dog, an egg-salad sandwich, and a sweet iced tea.
He was so habitual about his order that he could go
into the shop, stand at the counter, and they would
fill his order; he would pay, and never say a word.
Having witnessed this, one woman customer was
convinced that Wes was a deaf-mute. Far be it from
Wes to tell her any differently. He was just there to

have a great time, spend a few hours with his many friends, party with the boys, and see the ocean. He came back mentally stronger than he had left and was ready for his next adventure.

That Tuesday, I received another message from Charles Williams about the other Charlotte. In it he proclaimed that she was doing well. He said she was radiant, even glowing. Of course she'd been taking radiation treatments in another attempt to shrink or kill the tumor in her chest. But Charles was always trying to find the lighter side of the situation.

Playing to Charles's incessant sense of nonsense, I replied, "Miss Charlotte's always been radiant! If she's getting more so, I'm gonna need sunglasses just to be around her. She always did light up a room. By the way, Wes got to start his chemo today outpatient! Ain't that great? Sleeps in his own bed at night. Hooray! Somebody said they thought it was odd how I found excitement and happiness in my child being able to get his next round of chemo. It's like you say, you have to have a sense of humor and recognize that 'this too shall pass.' It's all so much better than the alternative."

Wes started his chemotherapy "in clinic" or, more properly, outpatient. We were looking forward to this development as it meant a scaling back of hospitalization.

Unfortunately, things don't always go as planned. Upon receiving the first round of chemo, Wes developed a rather high fever of 104.3 that night. After calling the doctor, we were instructed to bring him to the hospital for admission. We did so in the wee hours of the morning and spent the night on a floor unfamiliar with leukemia patients as the customary rooms were full. They did little for him during the night, and as Claire and I attempted to catch a few winks in the side chairs in the dark and tiny little room, we had a strange experience.

Wes, at one time, had developed a blood clot in his left arm during one attempt at using a PICC line. Since the nature and persistence of the clot was uncertain, no blood could be taken and no infusions given in the left arm. Upon admission, a sign was hung on his door and above the bed advising of the condition. About 2:00 AM a lab tech came in to take the blood samples ordered by the doctors. Leaving the room dark, with me half asleep, she put a tourniquet on his left arm. I awoke in time to stop her and advise her of the signage provided. It was obvious that she was encumbered by an attitude from something else as she barked, "I have a job to do!" She then punctured Wes's right arm with a needle that Wes described as being the size of a garden hose. For the first time in four months, Wes complained about his treatment. Previously compliant with all their requests, Wes never again allowed anyone to take blood without first inspecting the size of the needle. On future occasions, if the tech didn't have a light-blue butterfly needle on the cart, Wes would send them back to the lab to get one. I have no idea what set the tech's ship rocking that night, but she had no right to take it out on our son in his condition. Wounded physically and emotionally, Wes persevered. We prayed for a quick move to a floor where Wes's illness was recognized and his fragile nature respected. We went home for real sleep early the next morning. I continued to try to control the uncontrollable.

Despite our eventual move to 6E, the leukemia floor, and the excellent care received there, all were unsuccessful in determining the origin of his fever. Wes was depressed. We eventually managed to get him home and realized that there are times when you must take your care in your own hands and ask the unasked questions that seem to be shouting for answers.

The results of his stay were that no cause was determined for the fever. A suspicious blood culture was thought to be from contamination of the sample as opposed to bacterial. Nonetheless, during his stay, they administered a very potent antibiotic and that regimen was supposed to continue upon his return home through home infusion. Wes experienced severe histamine reactions to this medication if given as normally prescribed, so the drug had to be administered slowly, and he required premedication in order to handle the infusion. Suffice it to say, the premeds were timed for a shorter infusion time than the antibiotic. Upon completion of the antibiotic infusion, Wes experienced a reaction similar to the asthma he had as a kid and things were critical for a few minutes. Fortunately, Claire knew immediately what to do and gave Wes the antihistamine Benadryl. In a few minutes the symptoms subsided, but the event had scared Wes. Beyond the physical strain of the reaction, the worst part of the episode was that his spirits had been down Monday and early Tuesday, and by the end of the infusion, he had been about to recover emotionally. Then the adverse reaction literally sucked the breath out of him and his emotional recovery. Disparaged by his condition and his treatment, he cried.

Fortunately, the following day was a different story. I was determined to gain some control to see if I could help our son. We arrived at the clinic on time, had labs drawn, and I was able to stall infusion until we could see the doctors. I managed to appeal to their sense of reason and convince them that since no bacterial justification could be confirmed for continuing this harsh antibiotic to which Wes had such an unfavorable reaction, it should be discontinued. They eventually relented and provided a protocol that was much more patient friendly and should make life easier for a while for Wes and us. Though not totally out of the dumps, his attitude improved with the news. Who could blame him? I, on the other hand, felt that I had won some small victory.

With high temps, trips to the hospital, clinic trips, antibiotic reactions, and bouts of depression, we'd not had much opportunity to discuss the bone marrow transplant. That decision still lurked in the shadows.

Wes's asthmatic reactions had us worried. It didn't seem that the doctors had any idea what was causing them. Throughout my business career, I'd understood that people of average ability could be successful leaders if they surrounded themselves with people smarter than themselves. I always tried to do that. This series of events caused me to call on one of my friends I place in that category. While in college at the University of Georgia, I'd made the acquaintance of and developed a friendship with a premed student. We'd drifted in and out of each other's lives over the thirty-some years since, but he had gone on to a successful pharmaceutical career and had become a doctor of pharmacology (PharmD) and a dear friend.

I explained Wes's obvious asthmatic reaction to the neutrophil colony-stimulating growth-factor drug Leukine that was being administered and asked his advice. True to the profession, he initially responded with more questions than answers before stepping out on a limb.

"Has anyone said what bacterial infection Wes had previously, even though they could not culture anything at the time? Opportunistic infections are naturally the main problem given his decreased immune function secondary to the treatment regimens and disease state. Have you heard anything about MRSA and has he gotten Vancomycin in any of his regimens? Just curious. What was the latest word on any fungal infection?"

My response was emblematic of my frustration.

"The Vanco is kicking his butt and eating him up. That's what we've been having the problem with," I replied. "I didn't go into detail earlier, but they took two cultures when he entered the hospital: one from his arm and one from the catheter. Only one grew anything. They suspected contamination of the sample, so they drew two more the day he left, and we were told today that neither grew anything. They, therefore, believe that the fever was just a chemo fever caused commonly by Cytarabine and not a bacterial infection after all. Meanwhile, as cover, they blasted his butt with Vanco. It blasts his poor emaciated body, and then screws with his head. It's tough on him and torture on us to watch."

It's amazing what one can learn when he or she is forced into a situation where there is no choice and failure to learn and adapt could mean life or death. We had started using medical terms to describe medical conditions as if we actually knew what was going on. Fortunately for me, I only had to talk about it while Claire had to actu-

ally administer meds. Our mutual learning curves
were steep and unrelenting. Previously, when we
watched a TV show like *ER*, *House*, or one of the
other hospital dramas, we'd listen as the doctors
called out dosages of various antibiotics or chemo-
therapies and think, "Wow! They're smart!" Now,
when we watch the shows and they call out drugs
like Vancomycin or amphotericin, I think, "Better
premed with Benadryl and watch the infusion time
to prevent a reaction." I never wanted to be this
smart.

11

News of Miss Charlotte and Home Field Advantage

I t was often hard to recognize that anyone else was dealing with anything more difficult than we were. It was hard to realize that it wasn't all about us. Drawing into our problems, it seemed as if it was all about us, but then we got a call from someone who was having a more difficult time, and it snapped us back into reality. Charles Williams snapped me. Charles wrote:

> Man! This stuff is challenging to say the least. Charlotte has been through it! Had to have a tooth extracted . . . very challenging when your counts are out of whack (not a

very scientific term but very expressive in
this instance). Almost over that now, face is
still a bit swollen and yellow/blue . . . but
improving!

Dr. Langston and the Emory folks
aren't pleased with the long (five-week)
radiation plan the radiation oncologists in
Hawkinsville are following. It's taking way
too long. This week, they have all gotten
together and rearranged the schedule. Now,
we're doing "two a day" trips and will be
finished here next Wednesday. In fact, we
have to miss the second treatment next
Tuesday and be in Atlanta for the setup for
the total body irradiation (TBI) that will be
a part of the high-density chemo regimen
that now appears to be coming up around
the 21st of July, well ahead of our tentative
plans.

That should mean stem-cell transplant or
more accurately, infusion, to be completed
by month's end and the long, slow process
of recovery underway . . . anticipate a month
or so in the hospital with several weeks
(months) in clinic after that.

Also, since her sister is a ten out of ten match, the present plan is to give Charlotte a booster shot of her stem cells about two months after Charlotte receives her own. Now, that looks like maybe the end of September. That might add a while to the recovery and introduce graft versus host problems, but hey, that's concern for another day and time.

I could read between the lines to hear Charles's frustrations. Few, other than those going through it, know the challenges this type of situation presents. The tentative nature of our schedules can only be recognized by those with schedules equally as delicate.

I guess when we entered into this journey, we committed our lives to the Lord and Emory and must, therefore, get out of the way and let the healing continue. It's such a difficult thing to do sometimes, when things for which you prepared don't materialize and a new direction is not only suggested but mandated. I watched other patients and caregivers in the clinic and hospital going through this process, and they seemed to ask the dumbest questions about their care. I tended to ask myself, "How can they not know that?" But looking back, I sometimes think they got it right, and I got it all wrong. It could have been better to not know but just go. What we know today in these situations is often, and likely, proved wrong tomorrow. So we just deal with today. That is, if we intend to maintain our sanity.

As a result of self-diagnosing a problem with the help of my PharmD friend, I suggested to Wes's doctors that his tolerance for Leukine had run out, and they switched him to Neupogen, a similar drug, which he had used before without consequence. The allergic reactions stopped immediately, and Wes actually started feeling pretty good. In fact, he felt good enough to go out on a date with a girl he had recently met. Despite our delight in seeing him feel better, we had a hard time letting him go. We just wanted to keep him safe during times of exposure. His counts were not yet up, and he was susceptible to anything.

Nonetheless, what a great thing it was to see Wes feel well enough to consider a date. Wes never suffered from a self-esteem problem, even though the chemo and the disease continued to take their toll on his ravaged body. At times his six-feet-two-inch frame held only 102 pounds of weight. Fortunately, baggy clothes were the style. Early on, when he lost his hair and still felt well enough to drive his convertible, Wes had gotten a great tan. Despite his illness, he looked great. Later, this tan became a problem, a rather significant problem.

Vancomycin, or Vanco, the "big gun," the antibiotic that had given Wes so many problems in the past had another in store for him. One of the side effects of the drug is that it affects the nerve endings in the skin, and if there has been some recent sun damage, it will recreate and worsen the effect from inside out. The burning sensation Wes experienced on his arms was almost unbearable at times. The skin turned red, blistered up, and hurt. Anesthetic creams were gingerly administered and were of some help but only temporarily. For this reason, even now in July, Wes tended to wear long-sleeve shirts as he drove around with the top down and the music playing. Wes was, like his dad, somewhat of a control freak. He was fastidious in his dress and carried himself with self-confidence. Even in his emaciated form, he was determined to look cool regardless of the circumstances.

Though Wes's counts were in the basement, he felt good, had lots of energy, was in great spirits, and was exercising his sense of humor often and quite effectively. Since he could have caught anything at any time from anybody during this stage of his treatment, we should probably have insisted on keeping him under wraps, but when he seldom felt good for very long, we just had to rely on the antibiotics to keep him safe while he practiced being Wes.

We were scheduled to meet again with the bone marrow transplant doctor for a consultation on Tuesday afternoon. We had many questions—most that we didn't want to ask and many for which we didn't really think we wanted the answers. We hoped that if the news wasn't going to be good, it could at least be tolerable.

12

What Did You Say?

Tuesday was July the 13th, exactly five months from the day that Wes was originally diagnosed. We had a meeting scheduled with the bone marrow transplant doctor. We had the entire immediate family come to hear the news and to ask the questions that must have been running around in their heads. So fearful that I would not ask the right thing or that in my fear and excitement, I might forget to ask something I should, I made a list, a list of pointed questions that I felt held import. Claire didn't even want to hear the questions, much less the answers. I went to the meeting armed with the following barrage of questions, prepared to ask them all and write down the answers.

Questions for Dr. Langston

- What is the likelihood the chemo to date has cured him?
- What is the likelihood the leukemia will return?
- Do you have a match?
- How valid is the match?
- Do you suggest BMT?
- Would he be required to undergo total body irradiation?
- How many doses are involved in the high-dose chemo?
- How long does it take?
- How quickly would it take his counts down?
- How quickly after the chemo will he receive the stem cells?
- How many times will he receive stem cells?
- Is there a possibility that he might not survive the high-dose chemo?
- What is the possibility that the stem cells won't take?
- What can be done then?
- What is the possibility that the host versus graft might be fatal?

- What is the likelihood that it might be fairly minor?
- Will what he's had so far affect his ability to be a father and/or will the BMT affect it? If so, how? Will this still be his DNA?
- Should he decide to do it, how soon can the BMT be scheduled?
- Realistically, what is the recovery time when he can resume his school course work?
- We've heard that treatment takes about one hundred days and there's a requirement to be ten minutes from the hospital. Is Duluth close enough?
- What is the likelihood of the leukemia recurring if he chooses the BMT?
- What is the likelihood of the leukemia recurring if he chooses NOT to have a BMT?

Now, to my recollection we had only met Dr. Amelia Langston on one other occasion. We had a meeting with her the day that they took Wes down for the lung biopsy, had kept him NPO since midnight the night before, lost his chart, and then didn't even do the test due to his blood pressure being so low because of dehydration from being

NPO. Through no fault of her own, on that day, she had represented "the system," wanted to talk about the unpleasant topic of bone marrow transplantation, and Wes's mood did not have room for any more bad news. That having been the first and only discussion with Dr. Langston, none of us knew quite what to expect from her on this day, but due to the direct and dour manner the BMT had been laid out previously, we braced ourselves for the questions that would demand answers, none of which were preferable. We were about to get the surprise of our lives.

Dr. Langston said, "Wes, based on what we see from your previous bone marrow biopsies, you appear to be in remission. Given your age and overall health, there's a 40 percent chance that it won't come back, and if it does, it'll be a while. Forty percent is a relatively high number. Why don't we just take a 'wait and see' approach?"

Not understanding exactly what she meant and knowing that the purpose of the meeting was to discuss a bone marrow transplant, I asked, "So what does that mean with respect to the bone marrow transplant?"

To which Dr. Langston replied, "Let's wait and see."

I persisted, "How long until you'll know?"

"Let's wait and see how he does and if it comes back. It might not."

"Dr. Langston, are you saying that you're not recommending a bone marrow transplant?"

"Not at this time. Let's just wait and see. We still need to schedule one last bone marrow biopsy in about a week, but if it comes out clean, we'll just wait and see."

Collectively and individually, the family was stunned. For five arduous months we had been working toward preparing Wes for the only known cure for leukemia, a bone marrow transplant, and at five months to the day, his medical caregivers were not suggesting following through and, to a very slight degree, giving us veiled hope that he might already be cured.

Elated but confused, we sat and listened as Dr. Langston continued to give us our marching orders. Wes would continue with his current regimen, with another and last round of chemo in about a week. Upon recovering from that round, he would be monitored, at first monthly, with blood tests and bone marrow biopsies every six months, to see how he progressed. Provided those remained clear, they might stretch out his monitoring.

As to the fungal infection in his lungs, she suggested that we have that surgically excised upon his recovery from his last round of chemo. It might be possible that it could be done in a semiminimally invasive procedure with a three-to-four-week recovery time. He could then be scheduled to return to school in January.

Needless to say, Wes was elated, as were we. He called all his friends, as we did ours, and spread the news. As you might imagine, everyone was experiencing emotions ranging between stunned and elated. I don't think Wes's feet hit the floor all weekend, and he was on the move. Top down and on the road.

After returning to the clinic on Monday and finding that his platelets had recovered sufficiently that he could be released for a week, Wes left again for Savannah, his escape and home away from home, to visit his friends, furniture, and to see his new apartment. During his last hospitalization, Wes's roommate had found another apartment with a two-car garage and had moved all their belongings to the new "digs." Wes was excited about the opportunity to see his new place. He would then return home on Tuesday and was scheduled for a bone marrow biopsy on Wednesday. Barring any complications, Wes would then start his last round of chemo on Thursday, hopefully outpatient.

His release had provided a short window for Claire and me to get out of town, so we left that Thursday night for our place in Ponte Vedra. We, too, planned to return on Tuesday. Having been consistently tethered to the home front for so long, we felt a little funny about leaving. However, our justification was that we would be two hours closer to Wes in Ponte Vedra than we would have been in Atlanta. At least, that's the excuse we were using, so we stuck to it.

Our visit to our place in Florida was short but welcome. The weather cooperated, and Claire and I sat at the ocean's door with our feet in the sand staring almost comatose at the wonder of God. We had books to read, but I believe that we were so truly exhausted that one day we slept all day long.

We managed to reach Wes by cell phone periodically as he did us. It was somewhat ironic that, throughout his teenage years, as with most teenagers, Wes, though not reluctant to talk to us, just didn't seem to prioritize doing so. Now, I suppose that recognizing his illness and the fact that we had been with him every day for every issue for five straight months, he seemed to relish speaking with us. There was an apparent comfort level there for him as there was for us.

We did return on Tuesday, as did Wes, and we all showed up at Emory on Wednesday for his bone marrow biopsy. This test was more painful than some of the others due to those administering the test not recognizing or taking seriously Wes's stated need for more-than-average pain medication. They thought he was kidding when he told them the dosage they needed to administer to keep him comfortable was at least double the normal dose. They found out later that it was no joke. Wes was the unfortunate recipient of their disbelief. But as always, he mustered up more strength and courage than most more-mature patients could have done and persevered.

This was a time for good news. It wasn't just for us but for Charles and Charlotte Williams, as well. Charles wrote:

> Dr. Langston told us yesterday that
> Charlotte's stem cells are engrafting which

is a miracle, particularly at day eight since transplant. That means she is already beginning to produce her own stem cells which will create white cells and platelets.

What all that means is that she is really getting better.

In fact, they indicated she would be released from the hospital even as early as this weekend.

We have to remain in Atlanta for a week or so in clinic to make sure her counts come up and that there are no other problems (might see you there), and then we might be home for a few weeks. Can you imagine?!

Of course, she will be back and forth to Atlanta for clinic days for a while, and she will be preparing for the final part of this project. In September, they are planning to use her sister's stem cells, a ten out of ten match, and have Charlotte go through what they call a mini transplant. That's about the same as what she has just done with her own cells. The difference is that her sister's haven't been exposed to chemo. The theory is that the procedure will further enhance

Charlotte's immune system to preclude a recurrence of cancer.

There are serious risks associated with that process, but it is considered worth the risks for the benefits that can be achieved.

This is incredibly good news, and I just wanted to tell you and let you know how excited we are!

Expect the best.

This was great news. Charlotte Williams, the patient, was a beacon of success for Wes and us as we continued on our journey.

We, too, had good news, but, of course, it was tempered with the reality associated with our struggle.

As mentioned before, cancer patients do, indeed, live their lives in installments. They try to live normal lives between doctor's visits, yet become incredibly anxious awaiting test results. It seems to literally be survival by fits and starts. Emotions are sensitized beyond one's wildest imagination.

This was a crucial point for us. If this biopsy came back negative, Wes would then be able to move through this phase and on with his life. The results were not due back until Monday, so again we had to wait a weekend. To say the least, emotions were keen and the five days between Wednesday and Monday were tense, more tense than usual. My nerves and Claire's were on edge, and during that time, we tested each other's resolve by arguing about petty matters. That was unusual for us, but we chalked it up to the stress our life dished out.

Monday finally came, and we got the results. The bone marrow biopsy was negative. Wes started the first of his last six chemo treatments that day.

We had experienced an unbelievable struggle to get to this point. We were relieved and cautiously optimistic that we were due the good news we were receiving. This installment of our life was reaping the dividends that the effort had justified. We felt that our diligence had paid a reward.

13

FUOs and the UFO
That KOed NOPI

I can't begin to express our feelings during this time. The time was truly surreal. We felt that we had run a marathon, rounded a corner, and the finish line was right up ahead. It was within our sight, and the tape was within our grasp.

Wes, too, was elated. The relief that he felt was evident in his tone, in his mood, and even in the way he walked. He was happy. Truly happy.

We saw little of Wes that weekend as he spent most of his time gallivanting around town in his little rocket, top down, visiting everyone he knew to give them the good news. Celebrations were plentiful.

That was the happiest weekend any of us had had in more than six months. We prepared for Wes to begin his last round of chemotherapy the next week. It would be administered at the clinic, and if all went as planned, Wes might never have to spend another night in the hospital. How cool would that be?

We were hopeful that Wes would complete that last round of chemo and recovery unscathed. That was not to be the case. With his counts down, he received two units of blood on Thursday, and by the time we returned home, he was running a low-grade fever. We monitored it Thursday night, and it was still there on Friday morning. By Friday afternoon, it had risen to 103, so we called the doctor, and Wes was readmitted to Emory on Friday evening. It appears that leukemia is such a prevalent disease that no beds were available on the leukemia floor or the bone marrow transplant floor, so they secured him another tiny and dark little room on the solid-tissue transplant floor. The staff was pleasant and compassionate but lacked knowledge regarding leukemia patients, so it was up to us and Wes to assure that they gave him the proper meds in the proper dosages at the proper times with the proper premedication over the proper intervals to prevent adverse reactions. Surprisingly, they didn't often want to take the word of patients who had been dealing with the disease for six months over the word or advice of a resident who had never dealt with it. One nurse, not being familiar with the disease but understanding that leukemia patients could be infected by other germs, came into Wes's room wearing paper shoes, a paper gown, cap, mask, and gloves to take Wes's temperature. This guy was donned in full HAZMAT regalia like the EPA wears to clean up a hazardous environmental spill site. He walked in the room looking like the Michelin man. Claire looked at me, and I looked at her as if to say, "What's his deal?" To say the least, that was just another example of the challenges we continued to face.

Wes's temp stayed up in the 102 to 103 range as they administered fluids to prevent dehydration. Despite that, his mood was good and his sense of humor remained high. We had been hopeful that Monday his counts would have recovered to a point where he could finally be released, but this situation had created new concerns about the imminence of his release.

We were searching for answers to his feverish
state. It seemed that one minute we were on the
road to recovery and the next, we were back
in the hospital with tubes and lines running in
different directions. What would you do? Emory
couldn't seem to find the source of Wes's fever, so
I asked my PharmD friend if he'd ever heard of a
Vancomycin-induced fever.

You'll recall that Vanco was the drug that gave
Wes the red man syndrome if he was not properly
premedicated and that he had to take it at over at
least two and a half times the recommended dosage
time. It also seemed to blister his skin from the
inside out and just made him feel bad and mad. So
what did they do? They increased his dosage from
once every eleven hours to once every eight. Go
figure.

Every time I asked what I thought to be a fairly
straightforward question, my friend responded
with questions. His questions forced me to be more
clinical in my thinking. Therefore, I got back more
clinical information, but it was information that was
crucial at that point in Wes's treatment. This was
stuff I needed to know, and I felt blessed to have
a friend who had the answers that I needed. But

before I got the answers to mine, he had questions of his own.

"As we well knew by now, the red man syndrome is caused by too-rapid infusion of the Vancomycin. Wes sounds extremely sensitive in that it takes so long to infuse him. Have you heard anyone mention what his eosinophil counts are? I'm just taking stabs in the dark, but he could be running a fever just from a hypersensitivity reaction (in which case he may very well have an elevated eosinophil count).

"Has he also had shortness of breath associated with the Vanco infusions?

"I'm thinking that they continue the Vancomycin because they want to head off any possibility of methicillin-resistant staph.

"What is the latest news on the fungal lung mass? Is he continuing to get the antifungal agents via injection?"

The exchange continued as I tried to get some answers that I felt I might not be getting from Emory. I explained to him that they had done a full body scan the previous night. The abdomen looked good, but there was a curious area in the lung, different from what they had seen previously and not as well organized. They had him scheduled for a bronchoscopy the next day hoping that the results would identify the concern.

No shortness of breath had occurred during administration of the drug and no mention of eosinophil counts had ever been made (though I had no idea what they were).

I just wasn't getting the answers I needed and my ability to sit back and let somebody else control the situation was severely hampered by those people *not* controlling the situation or, at least, not fast enough for my tastes. So that night I delicately complained about them always finding this stuff on Friday night causing us to have two dead days in the hospital before any effective care was rendered to my sick son. Surprisingly, they then indicated an opportunity to do the test on Saturday. My concern was that they would pay him back by making him NPO after midnight and not getting to him until 4:00 PM. Been there. Done that.

The fact that a staph infection was mentioned was not lost on us. Wes had only started experiencing the fever after receiving blood at the clinic. Up to that point he'd been fine.

My friend responded to my questions in the following fashion.

"Eosinophils are a variation of white cell that proliferates in allergic reactions and it is not unusual for the counts to be elevated in Vancomycin hypersensitivity reactions. There are reports in the literature of fever of unknown origin (called FUO) occurring in association with Vanco use and appearing as much as five or more days following the infusions.

"The staph I mentioned is a gram+ bacteria that is especially nasty in the version known as MRSA or methicillin-resistant staph aureus. In fact, Vancomycin is the drug of choice in such situations. The inherent problem with MRSA out of control is that the bacteria release toxins and stimulate the body to produce a typical reaction which can result in sequences of events leading to problems such as abnormal blood coagulation among others.

"It doesn't sound as if Wes is involved with this type situation—but they want to make sure he doesn't become so. Keep in mind these are all guesses on my part."

His guesses were valued, and more times than not, exactly correct. They continually provided ammunition to use in assessing Wes's condition and treatment options. We were continually tested and confounded by maladies of unknown sources. FUOs? UFOs? They all started to take their toll.

Wes became somewhat depressed over the findings. He had anticipated being released on Monday of that week and to be in the hospital still was a significant psychological setback. He had little appetite due to the drugs and something had been irritating his eyes. Another scan was scheduled for the next day.

We were at our wits' end. It was extremely difficult to watch our child continually muster courage to face additional tests and more drug administration.

Uncertain of the source of the fever, the doctors made the assessment that the source, since the fever was not responding to antibiotics, must be fungal, and to top it off a fungus that didn't respond to the antifungal medication Wes was taking. They decided to try a new regimen. Then things got scary.

Though Wes's fever had abated somewhat since first admission, it remained above normal and his doctors were fervently searching for the cause. After a rather uneventful bronchoscopy in the morning, the afternoon was full of firsts for Wes and us.

First, the good news. Wes had developed conjunctivitis in his eyes a few days previous and though not painful, his eyes just looked terrible. The antibiotic they had prescribed for him seemed to be working to correct that malady.

His oncologist did change his drug regimen and prescribed two new drugs to replace two old ones. The first, imipenem, commonly referred to as "gorilla-pen" by those in the industry, is a strong, broad-based antibiotic. The second antifungal, amphotericin, was referred to by those who had dealt with it as "shake and bake" because the side effects were chills and fever.

Claire and I had gone to get a bite to eat that afternoon and left Brittany with Wes. Lunch was an opportunity for Claire and me to recharge our batteries, so to speak. We would take the elevator downstairs and walk out the back door of the hospital that leads to the Emory University campus. Once there, we could go to the student cafeteria where we could enjoy Chick-fil-A, Burger King, or a deli sandwich or salad. We would often walk to Emory Village and get a salad or pizza. At lunch we could decompress and share some time together and reconnect with each other. The stresses of the day seemed to disconnect us from each other, and it was at these times that we realized how much we depended on each other for strength and support. Lunch was a short respite in an otherwise hectic world.

Prior to our leaving for lunch, we watched as the nurses premedicated Wes in an attempt to ward off any allergic reaction to the drug, but while Britt and Wes were alone, Wes began shaking so violently, Brittany, stunned and confused, had to lie on top of Wes to keep him from convulsing off the bed. She screamed for help and finally the nurses came in and gave him Demerol to stop the reaction. To Britt it seemed interminable. It took three shots of Demerol before he calmed down. His reaction scared him and us, but especially scared Britt, bless her heart.

Reluctantly, we had to recognize that Wes was to have three more infusions of "shake and bake." We were assured that they would premedicate him with steroids prior to the infusion to prevent a reoccurrence. Based on previous track records with his allergic reactions, I can't say we were all that comforted by their assurances. We couldn't imagine the next day being any worse than this one.

We needed some relief. The stress and anticipation of each second and not knowing what to
expect were taking a toll on us. It was like that
joke about the guy up in the tree in a tussle with a
bobcat screaming to his friend with the rifle on the
ground to shoot. The friend, not being able to see
the wrestling movements stop long enough to get a
clear shot at the bobcat, was reluctant to fire. "Just
go ahead and shoot!" screamed the guy in the tree.
"One of us needs some relief."

After about three days, we finally started to
see some improvement. Wes was definitely better.
The fever had subsided, and they'd started stripping antibiotic infusions. He'd had a lung biopsy on
Tuesday. The bronchoscopy and the lung biopsy had
not yet grown anything from the cultures.

The medical staff believed the culprit to be
fungal. They anticipated releasing him on Friday
and continuing the amphotericin infusions for thirty
days with a weekend off the 17th so that he could
go to the NOPI Nationals in Hampton, Georgia,
where his cars had won the past two years.

Wes's attitude was improving as he could see
a way out. His appetite improved as well. We took
him two McDonald's cheeseburgers and fries for

lunch that day, and he ate both, as well as some brownies that Claire had baked.

As you can imagine, Wes, in an effort to take his mind off of his illness, was focused on his car and the trip to NOPI. He would have me write on the marker board in his room the items he intended to complete on his car between the time he got out of the hospital and the date of the show. Next to each item, he would quote a cost from memory, constantly asking me to total and retotal to be sure he could afford to make it look the best. Little did he know, and I didn't let on, but I'd have moved heaven and earth to do anything I could to make him happy. But he was in control of this. It seemed this was the first time he'd been in control of anything since February, so I felt it wiser to let him do it. I enjoyed seeing him excited.

Wes must have felt confused. My psyche wasn't feeling too good, and his must have been on life support. By now, he should be well. According to what he had been told by his doctors just two weeks before, he should be finished with his treatments and released by the doctors to resume his life again. Yet, for some strange reason, he found himself still in the hospital with some sort of mysterious

infection that confounded the doctors and continued
to tether him to the hospital, clinic, or home therapy.
He just couldn't catch a break. Little did he or we
know how literal that was about to be. But first, we
took time to exhale.

Wes did get home. They released him from
Emory that Friday afternoon after the CT scan in the
morning revealed that the fungal issue in his lung
had begun cavitation, the action of breaking up.
That was a good sign. The protocol going forward
was to return to the clinic each day for infusions
of the antifungal. After the reaction the first day,
they premedicated him with steroids for two days,
and after Wes experienced no reactions, they began
premedicating him with only Benadryl as his body
acclimated to the drug. These daily infusions and
oral antibiotics would continue for two weeks and
then they would do another CT scan to see what, if
anything, needed to continue being done.

He'd made plans to go to the University of
Georgia/Georgia Southern University football
game on Saturday in Statesboro, Georgia. He only
weighed about 114 pounds, so our task seemed
to be to fatten him up, if we could only slow him
down long enough to eat. Claire would make him

chocolate milk shakes with a raw egg, protein supplements, and a little vanilla extract. He loved them and would wolf them down until he had a brain freeze. He was so glad to be free; he was darting around in a blur.

The week continued to offer us some respite in the continued ordeal. We took those morsels and extrapolated them to yield a full recovery of Wes's condition in our minds. The hope accorded to his health gave our hearts room to beat. Some of the fear started to melt away.

As life would have it, this was the week of the hurricanes in Florida, and the storms impacted Ponte Vedra and our condo. Unable to leave town to check on it, we had to rely on third-party investigators to relay news and coordinate repair. We received a call from the company that provides caretaking services advising that water had blown in under the sliding glass doors and soaked the carpets. As well, we were told that the wallpaper was peeling in the master bedroom. When the insurance carrier was contacted, we were told, "You don't really want to make a claim, do you?" It was pretty apparent that making a claim on our policy could result in cancellation of coverage. Normally, this type of situation would have devastated us, but we just chuckled at the occurrence. We realized how material things couldn't have the same impact on your life that your loved ones can. It'd be okay. It was just stuff, and stuff can be fixed. But, you know, life really isn't fair.

I got a note from Charles Williams that week updating us on Charlotte's progress and treatment. He wrote:

Charlotte has a 9:00 clinic and then a 9:30 consent session with Dr. Langston for the upcoming allogeneic stem cell transplant. She is to be admitted this Thursday for chemo, round twelve, to suppress, not kill, her immune system in preparation for the infusion of her sister's stem cells. That is planned for Wednesday, the 22nd. Busy couple of weeks.

With all that completed, we expect to be released from the hospital in early October but be required to remain in the area, Chip's place, until around Christmas.

Expect nothing less than the best.

We'd become quite close to Charles and Charlotte Williams through a chain of events we both would have preferred to avoid. We needed them, and I hope we were able to add something positive to their lives as well.

To say the least, Wes was elated to be out and free for the weekend so that he could go to the NOPI Nationals in Hampton, Georgia. He was buzzing around town getting all the details handled to put his car atop the field of entrants he was bound to face. Wes, despite his weakened body, was up to the task in spirit and excitement. He had coordinated the trip with some of his best friends, and they were to leave for Hampton Thursday afternoon. They were to spend three nights there and return on Sunday after the competition. But as before, Wes just couldn't seem to catch a break. The Wednesday prior to NOPI was no exception.

Everything had been going fine at the clinic, and Wes was scheduled for a CT scan on Thursday afternoon that would hopefully show sufficient cavitation of the fungal mass to allow the doctor to release him on Friday. Though this was not certain by any means, it was our mutual hope.

Wes had been working furiously on his car each day after clinic trips to enter it in competition and attempt to win a trophy in his division for the third year in a row. He had coordinated installation of equipment by the minute between then and Friday night so that he could go down early Saturday morning and register for the competition. The devil was, however, in the details.

At about 3:00 PM we got a call from Wes. Fortunately, we were close by. Wes had had a wreck. It seemed that, between trips to suppliers, as Wes was entering an intersection, another driver turned left in front of him and collided with the left side of Wes's show car and, as best we could tell, totaled it. NOPI competition was now an impossibility and the "three-peat" couldn't happen. Wes was physically okay. The Honda S2000 held up superbly considering the impact. Both air bags deployed, but Wes was actually able to open his door and exit the vehicle. What a testament to Honda. If Wes had been going any faster, the guy would have hit him in the driver's door.

Wes, despite his devastation, was philosophical as evidenced by his comment when he said dejectedly, "Everything happens for a reason."

I was livid. Wes was being much more mature about it. I guess we all live long enough to learn from our kids. He seemed to be okay with the thought that the car was just stuff and unimportant in the big picture. He was still hurt by the dashing of his hard work. I hurt for him too.

We had the car towed to the Honda store for repair. They quoted Wes the obligatory thirty-day repair time and the at-fault driver's insurance company rented Wes a car to drive. It was a small econo-box with little style, little power, and no sex appeal. Wes seemed to take even this in stride despite the fact that I knew he was not in his element outside of his high-powered, high-attention, convertible rocket. He resigned it to fate and decided to go to NOPI anyway. Unfortunately, many of his friends bailed on him and decided not to go. Up to this point, NOPI had had somewhat of a party atmosphere, and Wes was looking forward to that aspect of the event. It was immediately evident that the party was not going to happen. So it was just Wes and another friend who went, to be joined later by one other. Not surprisingly, Wes didn't have much fun and came home early, depressed and just generally unhappy. His trip was probably analogous to the last time a teenager goes trick or treating for Halloween. You want it to be as fun as it always had been, but you've changed and that part of your personal history will never repeat itself. That ship had sailed.

Charlie Williams was counting on a ship sailing too. His was for a good reason, though. I could almost hear the excitement in his voice as I read his words.

> It's Monday morning and today should be, could be, hope and pray will be Charlotte's last day of chemo . . . EVER. The drugs are administered at night, around 11:00 PM till 12:30 AM. Tonight may well be the last in this long, long journey.
>
> Expect the best.

I knew of few people who deserved good news more than Charles and Charlotte. Charles continued to share good news and optimism three days later.

> Charlotte had a very good day. Her sister was able to collect 14,000,000-plus stem cells (that's a lot), and the Emory team was

able to infuse them into Charlotte. Two
major hurdles cleared.

Expect the best.

And we did expect the best for Charlotte and
continued to expect the best for Wes.

We rocked along for a week with this fungal
issue requiring daily trips to the clinic for Wes and
us. The following Monday, the doctor felt that we
could cut down the trips to three days a week for
the next three weeks with a CT scan scheduled at
the end of that time to determine if the mass had
shrunk. Previous scans had shown no change. It was
hypothesized that the mass had shrunk all it would.
Maybe that was a good thing. We were elated and
cautiously optimistic.

But then, as had been our experience, "Just
when we thought it was safe to go back in the water
. . ." Having our clinic visits cut back, we were
feeling good, Wes was tolerating the antifungal
medication well, and the doctor walked by and
casually mentioned, "We're picking up something
curious on the blood tests. Now, this shouldn't be
reason for concern because it could just be the antifungal. This stuff is poison and does strange things

to your system but, just to be on the safe side, since we haven't done one since the last round of chemo, let's schedule a bone marrow biopsy just to take a look and be sure there's no reason for concern."

We didn't waste any time. We had the bone marrow biopsy that afternoon and awaited the results on Wednesday. Despite the doctor's attempt at consolation that this shouldn't be reason for concern, we were, in fact, concerned. We were hopeful that these curious events were not a recurrence of the leukemia.

I tried to be strong under all the circumstances we faced. It was important for the family to have someone who had broad shoulders and could bear up under the pressure.

I tried valiantly to maintain a positive outlook but now even positive seemed to have its limitations. Honestly, my attitude sucked right then. I had felt an obligation, a duty, and a responsibility to keep my son healthy, to save him from this demon leukemia. This recovery was analogous to water torture. Up. Down. Up. Down. Up. Sideways. Down. Sideways. Up. Up. Down. Just about the time you thought you saw a light at the end of the tunnel, you'd seemingly hear a horn. Hopefully, it wouldn't be in our tunnel. I was fearful that I had failed in regard to Wes.

That morning before we went into the clinic, before we got out of the car, I asked Wes to pray with me. I'd never done that before, prayed one on one with any of my children, but Wes and I prayed that God would give us the strength to handle whatever news we got. We were beginning to understand how little we understood about God's will and that we should just trust Him and lean on Him for strength and comfort. I had significant difficulty with the entire concept. I was crumbling inside.

Listen! What was that noise? A horn?

That Wednesday we got the news that we feared. It was a horn and it was in our tunnel. It was back.

14

Raw Fear and
Searching for Support

I had been concerned since the mention by the doctor on Monday that there was something curious in the blood, and the feeling was reinforced by Wes's sniffles and his eyes. His counts came back at 28,000 and the results of the bone marrow biopsy taken that Monday confirmed that the leukemia was back. We knew from the first talk of release that there was only a 40 percent chance of success. So the 60 percent odds got us.

We were to check Wes into the hospital the following afternoon, and they would begin administering chemo that night. The plan would be to get the leukemia under control and attempt to perform a bone marrow transplant in about six weeks.

As disheartening as the news was to accept, God had apparently given Wes that peace that surpasses all understanding, and Wes actually told a friend on the phone that he felt good about this. I just hoped that Wes had the strength to tolerate the new round of chemo with the courage and fortitude he had in the past and prayed that the new regimen would produce the long-awaited cure for which we all hoped.

One would have thought that facing life without my dad—being left with a family business that was $1,000,000 in debt during an economic downturn with various skirmishes around the edges of bankruptcy and fear of losing our franchise and the entire dream my dad had embraced his whole life—would have prepared me for anything. For that reason, up to this point in my life, I was pretty sure that I'd known fear. Apparently, I was wrong.

I couldn't necessarily discuss my fear with the family. To do so might put their hope for Wes and his complete recovery at risk. I had to look elsewhere to find some comfort in sharing my emotions. I chose to contact my best friend again. This is how

I voiced my concern. To say more would have been emotionally impossible.

"Hey man, you know I love you and don't want my burden to become yours, but this is bad and I'm scared. We'll know more in a couple of days but I truly believe we need a miracle."

Poor guy. He simply didn't know how to respond. He simply and adequately promised his emotional support and fervent prayers for the miracle we sought.

Returning home from the hospital one night, the fear had ravaged my psyche to the point of total exhaustion. My lack of control had over-whelmed the "me" that I was. I didn't know who I was now. I was whipped. As a child, I'd grown up in the church. Claire and I had met there. After some young adult consternation, I'd even started going with some regularity, and then with extreme regularity. We'd raised our children in the church. But the efficacy of prayer had always eluded me. We said grace before meals, and I had previously tried to invoke God's help when things went south with my business. But from what I could tell, the prayers I sent up simply bounced off the ceiling. I had not felt God's hand in response to any prayer

I had offered. But with the degree of emotional devastation and fear we felt about Wes's situation that very second, I knew nowhere else to turn. That night, when we entered the house, I took Claire by the hand; we went in our sunroom, pulled out an ottoman, she on one side and me on the other. I pulled her down with me to our knees and there, with hands clasped together, heads resting on each other's shoulders, leaning all our weight on each other and that ottoman, I cried and prayed.

I beseeched God's mercy on Wes. I asked for understanding. I prayed for our other children. I prayed for the doctors. I prayed for God to reveal His will to me. I prayed for strength. And I prayed for peace for my emotionally ravaged soul.

I don't know how long I prayed or how long we stayed on our knees and cried together, but when we arose, we were cried out and physically exhausted.

I couldn't then and can't now remember the last time I was on my knees in prayer prior to that night. Previous episodes are likely to have been mere recitations. This night, I pled with God. I really prayed. As before, I waited to see God's hand. I was hopeful, even prayerful. My will had been insufficient. Perhaps His would be more effective.

As luck would have it, Wes's admission to
the hospital occurred at a time when his primary
oncologists were going out to San Diego to a
conference. Though this, in and of itself, could be
a good thing (should they hear of a clinical trial or
some new treatment on the horizon), it left us with
another new doctor. He was in his early to midforties, about five feet nine inches tall with a receding
hairline, wire-rimmed glasses, and a neatly trimmed
mustache and goatee. He wore a French-blue shirt
under his lab coat and a bow tie.

Dr. Waller was not truly a new doctor; he was
a seasoned leukemia researcher. We found out later
that his own son had been diagnosed with leukemia
some years prior, and this father had dedicated
himself to curing his son and to date had been
successful. We immediately liked him, his serious
yet calm demeanor and his direct approach. That
direct approach came early into our introduction
during his first session with Wes.

"Wes," the doctor said, "you could easily say
that you were tired of all this and decide to quit.
Frankly, the odds aren't in our favor, probably
somewhere in the 10 percent range, so if you'd

rather not endure any more of this chemotherapy, you just give me the word, and we'll stop."

To our delight and wonder, Wes replied, "Doctor, quitting is not an option."

The new plan was to attempt to control the leukemia and get it into remission with a one-time dose of a chemotherapy infused with monoclonal antibodies that would target the leukemia cells, attach to them, kill them, and shepherd them out of Wes's body. It was high-powered stuff and could cause significant difficulties with other organs as his kidneys and liver tried to process the chemo-therapy and the trashed cells it would create. They had to monitor those closely. Wes got that infusion on Friday. He tolerated it well. That was good. It would take two days for the results to fully manifest and for the counts to drop. They started dropping the following afternoon, and we believed that to be good. As the nurse said, "We need to keep them going in that direction." Wes's attitude was good despite not having his car or NOPI to maintain his focus. His appetite was improving. Those were good things. The hope was that the chemo would manage to get him into remission so that another bone marrow biopsy could be conducted in two weeks showing the blast cells gone. Wes could then begin immediately preparing for a stem cell transplant to provide a cure.

The scary part for us was the slim chance given for success in each step. Wes understood the odds and exhibited great courage with his perseverance.

I had continued to e-mail our friends each week, or when we would receive some news. I didn't want to become an unwelcome intrusion in their in-boxes but felt that they should know. After all, I had asked them to pray for Wes, and it seemed rude and insincere to request prayer from them and then estrange them from the results. I had an obligation to advise them, and it was easier to broadcast one e-mail message rather than repeat the same thing over and over in phone conversations with each one. What I came to realize was that our struggle had become fodder for further distribution over the Internet. The e-mails, my e-mails, were forwarded by others to others. For that reason the story of Wes's battle was heard far and wide. I received e-mails from strangers. People responded from as far away as Texas, New York, South Carolina, North Carolina, West Virginia, Washington State, Oregon, Florida, Alabama, London, Wales, and even Estonia. We found out in various and sundry ways. A neighbor e-mailed to explain how she came to hear about Wes again.

"I just returned home from a Christian women's retreat in Chattanooga, and our speaker shared with us that she had a list of people with cancer that she was praying for. She named Wes—no last name but she said he was twenty-two and had leukemia. I knew that it had to be your Wes. The speaker was Diane Parker. She was fantastic. Hope you receive much better news this week."

Diane had been a Sunday-school teacher of ours and many years ago had moved away and left our church. We hadn't spoken with her in years. We didn't even know that Diane knew of Wes's illness. The web is a powerful tool.

Charles Williams also kept in contact through e-mail as we did with him. We continually provided support for each other as we traveled down that cancerous road.

Still, Wes remained hospitalized, taking this new round of chemotherapy and the results, when graphed, appeared to make a sawtooth progression. They'd go down, then up, then down again, then up a little, then down, and so on. The overall direction was good, but we didn't know if this was normal or not. When we asked the doctor, we were told, "It's not uncommon to see this type of progression. Let's wait and see." Wes wasn't feeling the best, running low-grade fevers at night, experiencing some bone pain, significant nausea, and feeling generally crummy. However, the previous night there had been no fever, no nausea, and upon our arrival at the hospital that morning, Dr. Waller greeted us in the hall with the following words, "Counts continue to come down; I'm stripping away some of the fluids, and I want him out of the building for a while today. Take him to the museum over at Emory or some-where; get him out of the bed and out of here for a while." So we did.

As we left the hospital, we passed numerous patients outside smoking cigarettes while sitting in wheelchairs or tethered to IV poles. We said nothing but just looked at each other with a "why bother?" look and shook our collective heads.

We walked down to Emory Village and took Wes to Everybody's Pizza. He wasn't very hungry. After lunch, we walked back to the Michael C. Carlos Museum on the quadrangle of the Emory campus. Some years before, the Carlos Museum

was successful in making a bid for some rare
Egyptian artifacts. Included in those artifacts were
the sarcophagus of Rameses II and the mummy
of pharaoh Rameses I. Wes seemed to find the
museum interesting, and he tried very hard to be
lighthearted and humorous, but due to his tired
state, I think he would rather have welcomed his
bed. Nonetheless, Wes went slowly through the
museum, asking questions and making observa-
tions, though it was evident that it was tedious and
tiring for him. All in all, though, I think the outing
was good for him *and* us.

Wes's counts had been 84,000 when he was
admitted this time. They were now down to 19,000.
Complete remission would mean a count of zero.
We were just hopeful that his blood would coop-
erate with the chemotherapy so that his counts could
get into triple digits and we could take him home at
nights.

Claire and I were back in the routine of going
home at night to return the next morning. The trip
was so routine that we would see the same people
on the highway each day and wonder where they
were going. But the routine was not always so light-
hearted when it became apparent how our feelings

changed each morning when we arrived back at Emory. The road in front of the hospital was lined with imposing oak trees and the lanes narrowed. The congestion associated with a world-renowned hospital and a first-rate university created a swell of activity: traffic, buses, and pedestrians. The anticipation of not knowing what to expect of Wes or his condition would become so suffocating that it would literally suck the life out of our psychological selves. It made us want to be anywhere but there.

Three days later, we knew a little more, but only a precious little. The second half of Wes's week was better than the first. Though his counts had not come down as far or as fast as the doctors would have liked, the plan was for him to be released the next Monday to go home for home infusion of antibiotics and antifungals daily with clinic visits every other day and another infusion of the single-dose chemo on Thursday or Friday. That could be done in hospital or in clinic. That was not yet decided. Given that the next round of chemo might get his counts down to an acceptable level, preferably zero, he would then be monitored for a while prior to a stem cell transplant which we believed would happen within thirty days.

Other than a little nausea and a general malaise from the medications and illness, Wes's spirits remained pretty good. He was still a sick puppy. But his not feeling well was a blessing at times when his counts were down and he was so vulnerable to every kind of infection. If he'd felt better, he'd have been trying to get out and gallivant all over town; at least when he felt puny, he stayed put and protected.

The next few weeks were crucial. Claire and I could not worry Wes well, though we kept trying. We tried to lean solely on God for comfort during this storm. Yet we had to rely on the doctors and nurses at Emory to provide effective care for our son. Prayers were sent up asking for strength, for patience, for endurance, for understanding, and for peace. I know it sounds silly that I would even contemplate that there could be peace during this tumultuous time, but I had begun to find, since that night on the floor in our sunroom, that I was asking God for more and more help to deal with the events that continued to spiral out of my control.

One night, after returning home from the hospital, I was especially conflicted as I sat in the dark on our veranda. It felt as if my stomach, my heart, and my nerves were all jumbled up in a knot. I closed my eyes and prayed that God would provide the peace that surpasses all understanding. I knew it was a big order, but I'd had people quote the Scripture to me numerous times during Wes's illness. I somehow doubted the possibility that even God could find calm in this storm. Yet He did. Within about fifteen minutes of making that plea, I felt a sense of calm and warmth and peace come over me, and I realized that it could not have been of my own doing. It defied common sense. It was incomprehensible. It was that irrational peace that surpasses all understanding. Rather than God sending the lightning bolt I'd envisioned as a child or shaking me to the core, He made His presence known by just gently washing me in peace and love. I began to realize that this God was real. He heard my prayers and was there for me to lean on.

During the eighties, there was a television show entitled *ThirtySomething*. It starred Ken Olin, Timothy Busfield, and Patty Wettig. In it several friends who had grown up together reached their thirties and began to realize what adulthood was all about. On an Internet website the producers described it this way. "What they learned was that what they knew about life was enough to be totally confused by it."

TV shows rarely hold anything profound, but during the first season, one particular episode spoke volumes to me. Michael (Ken Olin) had been advised that his father was dying of brain cancer. He was standing outside the glass-enclosed ICU looking at his dad hooked up to all the monitors and IVs. As I recall the episode, his stepmother came to him and started asking a series of rapid-fire questions such as, "What should I do with the house? What about his life insurance? Who will handle the funeral arrangements? What will I do with my life? How can I go on?"

After that exchange, Michael stared into the room, and Hope, his wife, came over and Michael implored, "Hope, he can't die!"

"Michael," Hope said, "you heard the doctors; he can't live."

"But, Hope," Michael replied, "Don't you understand? I'm not ready to be the daddy."

With Wes in his current medical state, I wasn't ready for the responsibility of the decisions that loomed before me. I wasn't ready to be the daddy.

At that point, what I knew about life was that, like Michael, I was totally confused by it.

I needed more. I needed God to reveal Himself to me. I had to know that He was in control. And then it happened.

One Sunday morning while Wes was in the hospital, Claire and I were on our way to church just to "recharge our batteries" before going to the hospital for the day. We had been driving south on Interstate 85, not talking but listening to a religious music show on the radio. As my car came to a stop at the traffic light at the top of the exit ramp at Jimmy Carter Boulevard, Wayne Watson's song "For Such a Time as This" came on the radio, and he sang the line "I'll do Your will whatever it is . . ."

That was it! I had to be willing to do God's will, *whatever* it was. I had to let go. And I had to let God.

Claire had been praying for a miracle to cure Wes.

I had been praying for a miracle to cure Wes.

Everyone had been praying for a miracle to cure Wes.

What if that wasn't the miracle God had in store for Wes?

What if God—as in the Old Testament story in the Bible of Abraham surrendering Isaac to God—didn't really want Isaac? What if He really wanted Abraham? Maybe God wanted me. Maybe He wanted me to surrender Wes to Him.

I had thought that faith and trust were pretty much the same up until that moment in that car. They were practically interchangeable words. But in the clarity of that moment, it was revealed to me that they were and remained very different and distinct words.

Faith was what it took for Abraham to take Isaac up the mountain. Trust was what it took for Abraham to place him on the sacrificial altar. The difference was the step in between the two actions.

Surrender.

I had to surrender Wes to God and recognize that whatever God had in store for Wes, and us, was part of His plan, and we needed to accept the fact that He loved Wes and would not harm him.

Abraham's faithfulness—his willingness to surrender his only son—and the trust he placed in God enabled him to throw himself on the mercy of God and recognize His grace.

Could I be that faithful? Yes. I chose to believe that I could. I wasn't sure that I could, but it was the only thing I could do. I had to let God be God, not make Him my puppet or try to control Him. I couldn't be God. He was in charge.

At that traffic light at that second, I surrendered Wes to God. I surrendered control over Wes's health to God. I surrendered myself to God.

Amazingly, the inner conflict that had been waging within me for the past eight or nine months over trying to fix Wes came to an end. I recognized that Wes was in God's will, and I would try to do God's will, whatever it was.

15

The Faithfulness of Charles and the First "Talk"

Wes did make it home on Monday, and we started a home regimen. We tried to take it in stride. Wes had a good week. His attitude was good. Home represented family and safety to Wes and was the tether that kept him attached to this world. Often, in the late afternoon, we would find Wes in the grand room, sitting in a chair, looking out the window on its western exposure watching the sunset. The blues and oranges and pinks through the sky would paint a picture that changed with each few minutes but provided evidence to Wes that God was blessing him with strong and beautiful images even though he was physically weak.

He was moving around pretty well and liked being at home a lot better than being at the hospital. Originally, we were going to have to do four infusions per day over about six and a half hours. Fortunately, they changed one of the infusions to pill form so he had two infusions over two and a half hours. That worked pretty well. We went back to the clinic, and they infused him there and gave him platelets. We were to go back on Friday, suspecting Wes would need platelets again, to get his infusion and the doctors would consider giving him another round of chemo. His counts were continuing to come down but were not as clear as the doctors had hoped, so they felt another round was necessary to attempt to get him into a suitable condition for a stem cell transplant.

They started the buildup procedure on Monday with a CT scan and the scheduling of other tests necessary to prepare Wes for the stem cell transplant. If everything went according to plan, they anticipated doing the transplant in four to six weeks. We were prayerful that they would be able to get Wes to the point where that was possible. But first, more chemo.

The effects of chemotherapy are cumulative, and the reaction of one's body gets more severe with each round. This particular chemo treatment caused Wes to experience nausea, and he was unable to eat and felt generally lousy. If this was at all reminiscent of the last round, he would feel better the next day. There was some, but precious little, comfort in knowing what to expect. We learned to take control in whatever manner we were able.

Then we found that a precious little three-and-a-half-year-old girl in our church, had died as a result of a leukemia-like disease. She was so young but so wise and so courageous during her battle for life. How merciful was our God that she was spared further hardship. During her brief life, she provided a ministry to many demonstrating how to handle life as it's dealt with grace and charm. We recognized the family's grief over their loss but equally recognized how enriched heaven was by her sweet presence. Wes absorbed the news without comment.

She'd been a fighter, a three-year-old role model of courage, strength, and stamina for Wes and us to embrace. Her quiet and courageous struggle and her graceful passage to be with God were again an example of how an angel should deal with adversity and the trip home.

Then I heard from Charles Williams that they had received news that was not what they had hoped. A PET scan confirmed Charlotte's original tumor had increased in size over the previous PET study. The good news was the fact that it was not as bright on this scan as on the last. She was readmitted to the hospital that afternoon.

Despite this setback, her spirits were wonderful, a testament to the type of woman she was. She wasn't upset. Her faith was strong, and she was determined to meet the challenge one day at a time.

That night, Claire, Wes, and I prayed for Charles and Charlotte before dinner that God would grant them the strength, courage, and peace necessary to face this new challenge.

Charles was lucky to have a woman of such strong faith and conviction. I knew how important that was as Claire had exhibited the same type of faith and conviction as she went through breast cancer and now, as she dealt with Wes's illness.

Even then, in her distress, Charlotte's spirit was so bright that she was just a shining light. Charles, too, provided such a ministry to others with his positive outlook on life and his uplifting appraisals of everyone he met.

We'd both learned through this ordeal that for each two steps we took forward, there always seemed to be a step back. I was looking at this latest issue as merely a step back, and the next steps would be moving forward toward her complete cure.

Continued discussions with Charles indicated that he had a damaged spirit. It was obvious that he was disappointed with the new findings and scared for his lovely wife and himself, as we were for Wes and ourselves. The strength that God provided to each of us was an amazing thing. We didn't know how much we could endure until the hardship befell us. Then, miraculously, He stood by us as we struggled back to the top.

That endurance was foreshadowed in others we knew, who by example had shown us the path. So it was with a friend we'd met some fifteen years prior. A spectacular photorealistic artist of grand Southern mansions, seascapes, and human interest scenes, had been diagnosed with kidney cancer years ago and had been putting up a valiant fight against the *C* demon, this time with lung cancer. Having not heard from him in eight months, I decided to drop him a note. His reply stunned me. Apparently, he'd had a bout with pneumonia that slowed him down a little. Lots of antibiotics and chest X-rays. It seems that people who have had lung surgeries have a tendency for pneumonia, and he'd had both lungs operated on. His last surgery (his eighth) was in February in Washington DC where they removed tumors from his other lung. He'd had a set of scans and tests (MRI, CT scan, bone scan, etc.), and there were some suspicious spots on his remaining partial kidney that would require watching, but the doctors had said that he could consider himself stable for the imme- diate future. They were watching his blood tests; his hematocrit, platelets, and red blood count were all low, so he was extremely fatigued. He had more scans and tests in January of 2005. He was still doing some painting but not as much as in the past; he was unable to sit at the easel too long before backache set in as all of his back muscles had been cut several times and no longer functioned at 100 percent.

What an inspiration he had been to me during Wes's ordeal! Every time I hit a speed bump in the process, I'd think of him and the fact that he'd been through eight surgeries and had always had a deep faith in God and a positive outlook for all to see and witness. He had been a flag bearer for us.

Despite the inspiration provided to me throughout this episode in our life, I hadn't had an encouraging conversation with the doctor on Friday of that week and it put me in a position that seemed to be especially challenging.

The fungal infection persisted and the last round of chemo merely slowed the blast cells for a while. They were again on the rise.

Wes was unable to eat much, and his teeth and bones hurt, probably from the chemo.

We finally had a schedule for the bone marrow transplant (BMT). He would go into the hospital on September 18, begin receiving the strong chemo and total body irradiation immediately, and then receive the BMT on the 24th. He had to make it until the 24th.

Following the talk with the doctor on Friday, I approached Wes on Saturday morning as he was lying on the sofa in the sunroom. I had to have "the talk" with him. There were questions that needed to be answered, and I didn't feel right making those decisions for my adult son. He had to decide how much he would and could endure. It was one of the hardest things I'd ever had to do in my life. How do you talk to your own child about his mortality? I tried to do my best, despite my mentally exhausted state, to convince him that there is no dishonor in either decision. I tried unsuccessfully to hold back the tears as I asked him questions about whether he wanted to continue with the treatments. He remained somewhat stoic as I continued to ask questions regarding his resolve. I tried desperately not to make him think that we, or more specifically I, had given up on his recovery. He took it well. What courage.

Before you ask, yes, I'd searched for clinical trials elsewhere: at Johns Hopkins, the Mayo Clinic, the National Institute of Health, and M.D. Anderson. Wes had been ruled out of those few that applied due to having an active infection. I even called Hematology/BMT doctors at the Fred Hutchinson Cancer Research Center in Seattle and frantically spoke with them and was assured that everything that could be done was being done considering Wes's condition, the infection, the number of rounds of chemo he had received, and the toxicity associated with it. That was comforting to know, though it didn't make it any easier to see your child go through it.

Simply put, we needed a miracle.

The next twelve to eighteen days were extremely critical. I asked that our friends pray that God's will be done whatever that was. Despite our wishes, God's decisions are perfect in all respects. I was trying desperately to be as faithful as Abraham was with Isaac but it was just so hard.

Miracles were in short supply.

On Monday we found that Wes's disease was too active to continue on the transplant path. Both the leukemia and the fungal infection needed to be brought under control before he could be put back on the schedule. Neither cooperated.

The doctors at Emory had contacted the leukemia section at Northside Hospital, and they considered Wes for a clinical trial they were conducting. Again, Wes's active fungal infection ruled him out of the study. They said they would check further, and we would regroup on Wednesday to discuss other options.

Leukemia wouldn't wait until Wednesday.

16

A Scare at Home

On the heels of full recognition of the severity of the illness and the challenge of continued treatments, when we least expected it, another challenge grabbed us. An episode at the hospital clinic was one thing. When it happened at home, it was something altogether different.

Early in November, Sean and I were at home with Wes one afternoon while Claire was at Bible study. Wes had finished his infusion, was lying on the couch watching TV, and was in relatively good spirits when all of a sudden he started experiencing acute lower back pain. I have had two episodes with back pain and have some idea how excruciating it can be. I had never witnessed anyone in as much pain as Wes was exhibiting. I called his doctor and her PA, and they thought the pain was temporary and instructed me to give him additional pain pills. I did, and they did little to abate his pain. Preventing pain was much easier than easing it once it had developed.

I called Claire and asked her to come home. She did. Sean, having had some experience working at a hospital, remained calm and professional. He asked his mom to call 911 as he administered what aide he could to Wes. He then instructed Claire to go to the end of the driveway with her cell phone and await the ambulance so that she could direct it in. Then he instructed me to make a list of all of Wes's medications, the dosages, and the time when the last dose was taken. Initially, I thought Sean's instructions were analogous to the doctor in the old Western movies telling the husband of the pregnant bride in the ramshackle log cabin to go boil water just so that they could give him something to do and get him out of their hair. To the contrary, Sean's advice proved to be crucially important.

Meanwhile, in the midst of his pain and hardly able to speak, Wes whispered to Sean, "I sure do love you." That was Wes. Love was at his very core, and he expressed it freely despite his condition.

I did as Sean instructed and made a list of his medications, dosages, and times taken for the paramedics, in case Wes had to be admitted. He did. The paramedics put Wes on a gurney, loaded him in the ambulance, and took off for Gwinnett Medical Center. Though they obviously knew little about leukemia, the staff there knew about pain management, and within an hour or so Wes experienced relief to the point that he was, again, cracking jokes.

Upon our arrival, one of Claire's Bible study members, who had been visiting a sick friend in the hospital, met us at the emergency room. She had been called by another member of the Bible study. Soon, the emergency waiting room was filled with Claire's Bible study friends and husbands as well as her brother Robert, his wife, and three of their sons.

Only two of us were allowed in the emergency room with Wes at a time. Once, while I was in his room, a doctor Wes had never seen before approached Wes's bed with a vial of brown-colored liquid medication and was greeted by Wes's foolishness. Wes motioned to the bottle and then looked the doctor in the face and asked, "You back on the hard stuff again?" The doctor didn't know how to take Wes. Few did.

By about 7:30 PM Wes felt that he could stand
a car ride to Emory where a bed awaited him.
Now, a Mercedes is known for its smooth ride, but
the ride was more painful than Wes anticipated.
Despite riding in the back seat between Claire and
his cousin Josh, Wes felt the slightest road vibra-
tions, and they seemed to radiate through the seat
into his back. Eventually, we made it and about 9:15
PM he was admitted to 6E where, even at that late
hour, Dr. Winton came in and assured Wes he would
get him some relief for this continuing pain. After
mentioning that relief about three times, Wes asked
Dr. Winton if he could ask a question. Dr. Winton
said, "Sure!" to which Wes responded, "Could you
maybe get me that relief *now*?" Dr. Winton laughed
and immediately ordered the pain medication.

Wes liked pain medication and was one funny
person when he took it. By 11:00 PM with his pain
level about 40 percent of what it had been at its
peak, Wes's room was filled with his friends, and
Wes was sitting up in the bed demonstrating his ride
in the ambulance to their laughter. We felt it safe to
go home for the evening.

The following morning, we were advised that
they had found a regimen at another hospital that

had experienced about a 50 percent success rate in stabilizing relapsed AML leukemia patients. The regimen included a cocktail of three chemo drugs Wes had not taken. The idea was to stack these drugs in a manner to sneak up on and confuse the blast cells so that they were unable to mutate to become chemo resistant. Once they attempt to mutate to accommodate one chemo, they are hit with another, and by trying to mutate so quickly, when hit by the third, they die.

Options, at this late date, were becoming precious quantities. We'd been praying for a miracle, and we were praying that this was it. With new challenges came hope. Not a bright, shiny, strong hope like we'd had when Wes was first diagnosed but a weak, pallid, and slightly dimmed hope clouded by its unproductive brothers, fear and despair. Yes, we had a chance, but it was more and more evident that the chance cupboard was bare. This had to work.

"You don't know what you don't know." When a friend of mine first said that to me, I questioned his sanity until he explained its meaning. What we know of any situation is finite. This was true of leukemia, pain thresholds, auto mechanics, or nuclear physics. What we don't know about any of those topics is infinite. I had never realized this to be as true as it was at that moment.

Despite having no idea what the chemo was doing to the leukemia, we felt that the pain medication apparently worked well. Wes's friends found laughter in his antics, and Charles Williams came down to check on him in the midst of his "show." Charles remained an inspiration. Charlotte lay upstairs in a hospital bed with her own set of problems, and he took time to check on my kid. How amazing. I could not let that go unnoticed, so I e-mailed Charles.

> Thanks for the kind words about Wes.
> I would have hoped that Wes would have
> introduced his audience. My guess is that
> one was his brother, one was his sister, and
> one was his cousin. The others were a duke's
> mixture of his posse. He just surrounds
> himself with wonderful young friends, any
> of whom I'd be proud to call my own.
>
> Give Charlotte our love and remind
> her that more folks than she can possibly
> imagine are lifting her up daily. Sometimes

things seem bad because God wants to do something spectacular. His hand is on you both.

Charlotte was having a tough time of it. The doctors had told Charles that she had a low probability of survival. He was relying on his faith, and hers, to pull them through. We corresponded like brothers.

Charles, in recent days, I've been on the verge too. I could tell today, you were there. I'm sorry that the two of you are where you are, and I fully understand the incredible amount of strength it takes to just put one foot in front of the other. The weight of the world is on your shoulders. It's incredibly heavy. Just try to recognize that, though I can't physically do anything to alleviate Charlotte's discomfort or medically heal her, in spirit I'm under that world with you, pushing as hard as I can to lift and give you some breathing room. God's will is perfect in all respects. It may not be ours, but His is manifest in the world and the everlasting.

Unless some true miracle takes place,
I'll be where you are again. In those times
the two most important things to pray for are
that God's will be done and that you'll have
the peace that He promises us that surpasses
all understanding. He brought us together
for a reason. I'm convinced.

Wes continued in the hospital experiencing ups and downs. He continued his stay at Emory in an effort to get the leukemia under control, keep the fungus at bay, and alleviate the pain episodes. His counts were dropping, so we believed the chemo was doing what it was supposed to do. He had another pain episode on Wednesday and one on Thursday. Both occurred at about the same time, 2:45 PM, coincident with his antifungal infusion. Again, one happened while Brittany was alone with him. Once again, he shook so violently that she lay down on top of him to try to calm him. It was traumatic for him and probably equally traumatic for her. How was it that these episodes always seemed to happen when the two of them were alone?

Though the doctors had never seen a reaction to the antifungal like that, upon my questioning the coincidence, they switched him to another agent and changed the time, and he experienced no further pain episodes. Praise God. Now, the question remained, would this antifungal agent be as effective at fighting the fungus as the last? We had to wait and see.

Though he had no pain the next day, I think the chemo kicked his butt pretty good. He slept most of the day and didn't have any appetite. We were hopeful that it would improve the next day.

Just then, we were in a holding pattern to await the results of the chemotherapy regimen and were praying that it continued to be effective. We would know more later that week.

A friend of Sean's who worked for the Atlanta Falcons' football team came by to visit Wes, bringing Falcon team wear and good wishes. While there, he dialed his cell phone and handed it to Wes. On the phone was then Head Coach Jim Mora. He gave Wes a rather peppery pep talk and encouraged him to never give up. Wes was emboldened by his conversation.

Later, a neighborhood friend came by and brought Wes architectural books and car magazines. They shared conversation about mutual friends and Wes's plans when he got well.

As with all hospitals, scheduling requires shifting staff from time to time. One such shift introduced Wes to a nurse from a special hall at Emory that caters to wealthier patients. To begin with I think Wes was predisposed not to like her. I don't know why other than she was a more mature woman and was taking the place of one of the regular "hotties," as Wes referred to them. Despite Wes's initial attitude, she took to Wes right away. She told him that on this special wing, patients have a suite, their own private nurse, other amenities not afforded the typical hospital patient, and a chef to prepare whatever their taste buds and imaginations could conjure up.

One afternoon, as she was explaining this "celebrity" wing to Wes, she alluded to the chef and special meals. I could see after she left the room that Wes was scheming and putting a plan together. Sure enough, when she returned, Wes placed an order for a T-Bone, medium rare, a baked potato, and a salad with Thousand Island dressing. Laughing, she exited the room.

A little while later, she came back in, walked up to the head of Wes's bed, and asked, "Mr. Smith, what time would you like your steak delivered?"

Wes said, "Are you serious?"

She then confided that the special wing was empty, and it wouldn't hurt to put the chef to work. He was going to be there anyway.

And so, Wes had his T-bone and ate every bit, feeling much the celebrity himself.

Claire and I were thankful for her sweet and generous spirit and all the folks at Emory. They seemed to make a twenty-two-year-old with leukemia feel special every day.

As well, we were thankful for our friends' continued prayers on the behalf of Wes. He, too, was appreciative beyond measure. He knew what they were doing for him and continued to be in awe of their overwhelming love and support. Someone quoted a minister that week who'd said, "Never does one show that they love you more than when they pray for you." I believed that.

The routine swallowed us up so that one day ran into the next, and the change was gradual. Sometimes we got surprises and had to be careful not to allow the surprises to give us false hope.

Occasionally, we'd have that rare but good day.

Though Wes's week had been full of ups and downs (i.e., only minor pain, some fevers, mild nausea, etc.), one particular morning he awoke at 7:30 AM and walked about three-fourths of a mile around the hall; his fever was down, he was hungry, and we walked in to find him sitting on the side of his bed talking to a friend, alert, coherent, and feeling good about feeling good. Then the doctor came in and told us that the white count was down further (to 1,100 and that was a good thing), and the CT scan performed on Friday showed some improvement in the fungal mass despite having to change antifungal agents.

We simply took it one day at a time. We prayed now for another good day tomorrow and thanked the Lord for it.

Thanks seemed indeed appropriate considering that Thanksgiving Day was Thursday of that week. It only seemed proper that we thank those who had been so unrelentingly strong during the year. I tried to do so with the following words:

> I just wanted to take a moment to send a note of thanks to each and every one of you for your stalwart prayerfulness during Wes's illness this year.

Tomorrow, as we sit down to have our Thanksgiving meal, we have much for which to be thankful.

We have managed to get Wes a "day pass" from the hospital. He can leave at 9:00 AM, if he comes back by 6:00 PM. Provided that he has no fever and the staff at Emory allows him to come home for the day, we will be extremely thankful to have our family together for the meal.

Sean and Brittany have been so supportive and helpful during Wes's illness; we are thankful for the love they show us and each other.

Likewise, we are thankful for our families and extended families that have provided continued love and support throughout Wes's hospitalization and struggle with this dreaded disease.

Wes's friends have been vigilant in their visitation and expressions of love and support. Hardly a day goes by that one, two, or ten of his friends don't show up bearing gifts, good tidings, nonsense, or just companionship. How blessed Wes is to have such friends.

And that goes double for us. As we bow our heads tomorrow, we will give special thanks for each of you. We fully recognize how hectic life can be and that each of you has your own life, your own trials, and your own priorities. The fact that you can take the time to pray for Wes or us at any time just takes my breath away. We are deeply thankful for your sacrifice.

Lastly, we are thankful for our God who loved us enough to sacrifice His Son so that whatever we do, whatever happens in this life is going to be okay and we are guaranteed that He will never leave us or forsake us and will assure us of everlasting life. How great is that? What an example He sets for us. I will continue to pray that I am up to the task.

Thank you all for everything you do for us and mean to us.

Each day is so special. Each one is so different, as is each soul that God puts on this earth. Despite our differences, it had become apparent that God's love for us was the common denominator. When we all gather under that umbrella, we collectively generate a power that we lack individually. We continued to be thankful to those who were part of that powerful and prayerful force that exhibited God's love in such an unselfish manner.

I've heard it said, "Be careful what you ask for, you just might get it." We asked for a day pass for Wes to come home for Thanksgiving. He did get home, eventually. The results were less than optimum.

His 8:30 AM release was postponed until 10:45 PM due to a need for platelets and blood. The trip wore him out, but he did manage to sit at the table for a couple of hours and nibble on some turkey and the fixings. His car was finally out of the shop, and since this was the first time he'd seen it, he managed to drive it around the block, though he quickly recognized that his reaction time was not what it had been prior to the accident. When all was said and done and it was time to return to the hospital, it was painful for us to recognize that he was ready to go. It is incredibly difficult to realize that your child knows that he is too sick to be at home.

Once he returned to the hospital, Wes's counts started bouncing around in the mid 100s (500–800), and the blasts were still present. We prayed that the treatments he had received would take hold and alleviate the blast population so that he could begin recovery toward a stem cell transplant. We were hoping God had something spectacular in mind for Wes.

17

Larry's Chair

Once "back home" in his hospital room, Wes seemed to improve. His attitude was amazing, and he seemed more in his element.

When Wes felt good, and sometimes when he didn't, he seemed to be driven to help others. The community that develops from the twenty-five or so rooms on 6E, the leukemia hall, can become quite cohesive. Patients like Wes see to that. They tend to connect with the other patients. One such patient was Larry.

Larry was in his early thirties, married, and had something other than leukemia. He was a big guy but a gentle sort who walked the halls as instructed with relentless obsession. Wes met Larry while both were walking in the halls of 6E.

Soon they were visiting each other, supporting each other as best they could, considering their own conditions. After all the visitors of the day had left, Wes would slip down to Larry's room, and the two would talk and play video games until the wee hours of the morning. They forged a fast friendship.

When Larry was released just before Christmas of 2004, he "willed" two things to Wes that Wes had seen in Larry's room. The day of Larry's departure, the items were delivered by Wes's favorite nurse tech.

She was a grandmother, small in stature but huge in caring. She loved Wes, and it was evident in her dealings with him. During her off hours, she attended nursing school so she could eventually treat patients completely and render the care she felt in her heart.

She delivered Larry's bounty. One gift was a small artificial Christmas tree adorned with little boxing gloves that had been given to Larry by his grandmother. Wes was thrilled.

The other item was a huge leather recliner. Here was this nurse tech, this little ball of good will, shoving this huge chair down the hall from halfway around the floor. She muscled this mammoth blue chair into Wes's room that was already replete with two side chairs.

"What are you doing?" Claire asked.

Breathing hard, the tech said, "Wes wants it. Larry wanted him to have it. It's going in here. I don't care if one of those other chairs has to go out that window over there, he's gonna have this chair."

And so it was. Wes had his blue leather recliner. He would get out of bed, reposition his IV pole, and just sit in Larry's chair. That chair was sacred. Despite the fact that the other chair never went out the window after all, everyone dealt with "the chair"; the doctors, the nurses, the techs, family and friends. The chair made Wes happy and made him feel closer to Larry.

I don't know to what degree the chair had any effect, but all in all, Wes had a very good week. His counts dropped to the low 100s (400 being the lowest), and his blast count dropped to 24 percent (the lowest since the relapse). The doctors even talked about getting him out of the hospital. What a difference a couple of weeks made.

His lungs seemed clearer than they had in quite some time. They did another CT scan on Thursday and found no change since the CT of the 19th. We were hoping for better news. His appetite had come back, and his doctor made the comment that Wes was probably the only patient on the floor who wanted and ate barbecue. His attitude was superb. He'd walk often, meeting other patients on the floor and counseling them on procedures they were having done which he'd had done a while back, allaying their fears and assisting the nurses with the attitudinal problems some of the patients were exhibiting. The staff had formed a Wes fan club. Even a new female doctor, who seemed somewhat of a dour sort, lit up when somebody mentioned Wes's name. Staff from the BMT floor, the infusion center, PAs, patient coordinators, and off-duty nurses stopped by for regular visitation or called on the phone just to see how he was doing. It was amazing. I tried to be cautious but felt more optimistic than I had in quite some time. With his gentle spirit, genuine concern, and mild demeanor, Wes appeared to have been given some work from God, and we continued to pray that God had *much more* work for Wes to do.

Then, as we reveled in Wes's mission efforts, on December 5th we received this note from Charles.

I am delighted to tell you that my Charlotte is at this moment in heaven. She was fortunate to leave this world on Saturday, December 2nd at 4:40 PM. She left peacefully from her home in the warm hands and prayers of her immediate and close family.

Her illness was a blessing as it brought us closer together than ever before in our lives.

Thanks to our youngest son, Clint, and our outstanding business associates, our time together for this year and two months has been virtually uninterrupted.

Thanks to our oldest son, Chip, we had a comfortable home in Atlanta when we were not hospitalized.

Thanks to both of our closest family members, we were and continue to be surrounded by prayer and support. Charlotte's mom, her two sisters and their families have kept us close and strong throughout this ordeal.

Our wide circle of friends, especially those from Walton County (all twenty-four of them), and so many other friends and associates from around the state and across the country have brought happiness and encouragement through cards and e-mails and visits. This really is a wonderful world. It isn't perfect, but there is joy where you look for it.

Charlotte said from the first sign of her cancer, quite resolutely, that if she was allowed to live on in this world, that would be a dream come true, but should she leave this place and go to heaven, that would be even better.

The doctors and staff at Emory University hospital's oncology area were nothing less than extraordinary. It just was not to be. To name them all would take pages, but one nurse from our hometown— gave us every advantage. She is a dear and outstanding healthcare professional.

Charlotte's funeral service will be held in the First Baptist Church of Eastman on

Monday at 2:00 PM with two of our favorite people presiding, Dr. Jerry Peele, our pastor, and Dr. David Smith, our former youth minister and dear, dear friend from Austin, Texas. Judge George J. Hearn, III, will share memories.

Charlotte planned her service and will be honored by those who come and those who pray.

Please know our family is fine and loves you and your family. We wish you, Wes, and your family the very best in the upcoming holiday season. We love you dearly.

Charles

We had watched closely as Charlotte struggled with her illness and continued to see a picture of grace and charm uncommon in sick people. It was hard to believe when we saw her sweet smile that she really was sick. It was even harder now to think that she was gone.

That night, after receiving the word from Charles, I was conflicted with emotions. At one stage, my heart ached for Charles and the boys over their loss. At another, I was elated for Charlotte as she spent her first carefree day in quite some time and got to spend some time with her dad in heaven after a few months without him. I knew that Charles too was conflicted with emotions right then and offered a piece of advice given by my minister some twenty-two years ago when I lost my dad.

Right now, your emotions are raging all over the place. You feel them all. You experience grief, relief, pain, elation, sorrow, giddiness, tears and laughter, guilt and complacency, and it's scary how closely some of these are related. You, of course, feel grief over your loss but relief for her lack of suffering. In the height of your sorrow and tears, somebody recalls something so funny you laugh uncontrollably, and then you feel guilt for laughing when it is such a serious time. Rejoice and recognize that each and every emotion was given to you by a God who loves you deeply. They are genuine, they are valid, and He expects you to express them all. To do less would be shortchanging His wonderful gifts.

We all loved Charlotte. From those who had known her all her life to folks like us who knew her but just a brief time, she provided a light in our lives, and I'm sure that heaven is brighter by her presence. She had worked all her life to get to the podium, and she had finally graduated. What a triumph for her. I rejoiced at her success.

Somehow, we managed to tell Wes. He didn't seem shocked. He was pensive, introspective. He just kind of nodded a gentle acceptance. I don't recall either of us ever mentioning it again.

Regrettably, due to our concerns for Wes and our perceived need to be close by, we were unable to attend Miss Charlotte's funeral. Had we tried to, I don't know that I would have been strong enough to maintain my composure. Our love and bond had grown so deep, and we had shared a place at that table of hope and recovery. One leg was now missing from that table. Nonetheless, we persevered with Wes and things seemed to improve.

Wes came home again on the 8th. He felt pretty good and that was bolstered by a report that his white count was 500 and the blast cell count was 19 percent (the lowest it had been since the relapse). He got platelets before leaving the hospital, and they should hold through the next day. We were to return to the clinic on Friday for a consultation with the doctor regarding what steps, if any, would be taken next. The hardest part of this ordeal was watching your child go through it. The next hardest part was not knowing from day to day what to expect or even hope for. The doctors from the clinic had just returned from a symposium in San Diego, and Wes was to be a topic for discussion on Thursday at their meeting. We were hopeful that they had a game plan that would generate a successful outcome. We would see.

Friday came and the message was of clouded hope and encouragement. We were advised that Wes's last round of chemo had provided some wiggle room to explore other treatment options, mainly, clinical trials at other hospitals (M.D. Anderson, NIH, Mayo, etc.), if he qualified. He would likely still be excluded from those trials due to what was perceived to be an active fungal infection. We didn't get an accurate count on the blasts Friday, so we didn't know whether he was continuing to improve or regressing. Sometimes, not knowing was preferable to knowing. I guessed we'd find out on Monday. After a double dose of platelets, the doctors gave Wes (and us) the weekend off. Wes visited with friends each day, trying to be as normal as possible. With his counts so low, we still cringed at his potential bacterial exposure to others but figured he was on heavy-enough antibiotics and antifungals that, with reasonable amounts of hand washing, he could prevent most problems, if he exercised good judgment by staying away from obviously sick people.

So we were in what the doctor called a wait-and-see posture. Whether Wes's counts could recover without the blasts being present was the question.

Our cloud of hope and encouragement was "wait and see." It turned into wait and wait and wait. We had expected to have a meeting with the doctor to give us some direction on Monday or Wednesday. They put us off until the next Monday.

The bad news was that the blast cells appeared to be on the move again.

The good news was that the doctor we trusted the most and in whom we had the most confidence was apparently back on the case preparing a plan of attack. The other good news was Wes in general. His attitude was great. His sense of humor was nonstop, a real wise guy. He was doing stuff with his friends and being extremely careful to stay clear of anyone who was obviously sick, and he did a lot of hand sanitizing in the process. His appetite was great and other than some rather significant neuropathy in his feet that caused a burning and bruised feeling, he was doing okay, considering that he had leukemia. His platelets looked fairly strong and should hold through the weekend, so he had two free days over the weekend. We knew the disease was real. We had our doubts about our hope for Wes's recovery being real.

What was real was our need for continued prayer for Wes and his condition.

I'm pretty sure Wes had some question regarding the reality of a recovery. Upon being discharged back on the 8th, unknown to us, Wes pulled Keisha, one of his favorite nurses, to the side and asked, "Keisha, why are they releasing me with 19 percent blasts?"

Keisha gravely replied, "Wes, you'll have to ask the doctors."

And so it was that Wes, armed with that new bit of unspoken knowledge, headed home to experience a little well-deserved freedom.

We didn't know what to expect on Monday but reveled in the freedom of the next two days and watched Wes enjoy it as well. If he questioned the outcome, he did not show it.

18

Another "Talk" with a Lopsided Chipmunk

We did meet with the doctor on Monday and confirmed that Wes's blast counts had risen and were again approaching critical levels, so they started him on a maintenance chemotherapy regimen to attempt to bring those counts down over the holidays. It was the intent that this would be done outpatient at the clinic each day, and we were prayerful that Wes would be tolerant of this additional chemotherapy and that the neuropathy he had been experiencing would subside. No hope remained for the bone marrow transplant unless the leukemia could be brought under control. Previous chemotherapy had been unsuccessful in accomplishing that end. The plan was to devise yet another chemotherapy regimen to begin in hospital after the first of the year. Poor baby. I wondered how much his body could take.

Barring any unforeseen circumstances, we would be together for Christmas. With critical issues looming, it was quite difficult to be festive. Nonetheless, we were deeply appreciative of the support provided to the Smith family during the year by those who had known us for years and by those we'd just met. When we seemed least able to handle another bit of bad news, those friends were the knot in the end of our emotional rope. Claire and I continued to receive phone calls, e-mails, cards, and letters from those who expressed their love and concern to Wes and us. We had no idea what we would have done or become without them.

Christmas was different.

Wes got home for the holidays on Christmas Eve about 4:00 PM.

Christmas Eve was quiet as we chose to forego the customary Christmas Eve candlelight church service in deference to his susceptibility to catch a cold or the flu when exposed to crowds. Christmas Day, my mother and Sean and Brittany came over, and we exchanged gifts and had a big lunch. Wes's spirits were good. Christmas night, we again chose to forego tradition, and Wes and I stayed home while the rest of the family went to Claire's parents' house. Several relatives had been ill recently, and we didn't want to expose Wes, plus, I'd been battling a cold myself and didn't want to expose them. I could control my exposure to Wes (masks, changing rooms, hand washing, etc.) better in our own environment than when we were elsewhere. He and I had a good, quiet evening together.

Christmas Day was very different for us. The focus was on things other than tradition and the "way it's always been." Christmas marked the beginning of hope for mankind, and we still cling to that hope and the miracles that are evident within the story. God is a supernatural God and can do things outside this world through miracles that we witness each and every day. We continued to pray in that regard for Wes if a miracle of healing was His will. We had been blessed this Christmas by having Wes home, by sharing our food and faith and gifts with each other, and by counting our friends and family as part of our many blessings.

The New Year dawned with new meaning. I don't think I'd ever looked at the occasion in quite the same way. Despite our having our traditional guests for dinner and our attempts to be light-hearted, it was more a solemn event than a festive one. It was serious in all respects.

Wes's trip home for the holidays had been good, if uneventful. The last round of chemo seemed to arrest the development of additional blast cells and even caused them to abate somewhat. We still needed the miracle of having them disappear completely. With the New Year we had renewed hope. Wes's actions seemed to belie his illness. Though thin and pale and hampered by the neuropathy in his feet, his spirits remained high and his sense of humor sensitized beyond anything of which I'm capable. He had about fifteen of his friends over for New Year's. They were a compassionate and caring bunch, catering to Wes's needs while he tried fairly successfully to play the host through the apparent pain. Our emotions were in contrast as we watched the scene unfold.

We were to go back to the clinic on Monday for platelets and to see the doctor. Those were visits of contrast as well. We wanted to know, yet we didn't.

We needed the good news but seldom got any that would give us encouragement past the next couple of days when we'd do it all over again. It was a day-to-day thing.

Fortunately, Wes remained out of the hospital with periodically scheduled clinic visits. Other than Wes's developing a staph infection in a lymph node in his right cheek that made him resemble a lopsided chipmunk, that week had been seemingly uneventful. We'd seen the doctors a couple of times, and they'd told us nothing, good or bad. But that was sometimes preferred. The infection required two more daily infusions, Benadryl and Vancomycin, in addition to the antifungal caspofungin that he'd already been getting, and added another couple of hours to his down time each day. But he was bearing up well and taking it all in stride. The neuropathic pain in his feet continued, and the doctors continued to increase and amend the pain medication to see if they could make it tolerable for him. Wes persevered through the pain.

In many cases no news was good news. I couldn't be so sure in this situation. We'd gotten no blast counts from the doctors in a week, and though on Friday of the previous week, they had been in the high 20 percent category, I tended to think that if they were continuing to drop significantly, that would have made the news. Past history would indicate that some change was imminent within the next week or so. Wes had told the doctor at yesterday's meeting, "Just keep me out of the hospital; I've got things to do."

He did have things to do, and we wanted to help him do them.

The news that we hadn't been getting, we finally got, and, as expected, it wasn't good. The blasts were back. Though Wes's white count was relatively low, it was primarily made up of blast cells. That was not good.

That Sunday, Wes's doctors began the chemo regimen they had done the last time. In and of itself, we knew it was not a cure. It was simply to get him in a condition to prevent some of the more painful episodic situations that could occur with the disease as the counts escalated. It weakened him to endure it. He persevered in spite of it. What a guy!

Claire and I had painfully come to recognize that there are certain conditions with which man and medicine are not equipped to deal. God alone held the answer to Wes's disease.

We struggled each day with what is and isn't God's will. We believed that we could truly do it if we knew it, if it were up to us. We simply didn't know.

I found that praying for the peace that surpasses all understanding is different from just praying for peace. It's a different level of peace. By asking specifically for what you need, God delivers. It's like a cloud envelopes your entire body. It's pretty amazing. God is good.

As much as I hated to admit it, God was solely in control, not me. Nothing that I could consciously do would change any part of the outcome. So it was necessary to do some things that were simply peripheral to the outcome.

Wes had been a pretty frugal, hardworking kid. In being so, he had amassed quite a nice nest egg for a young man. He had IRAs, CDs, investment accounts, savings accounts, checking accounts, good credit, and a credit card account. But at that point, Wes was sick. Some arrangements needed to be made for those accounts. Trust me. I knew then, and I know now that it is much, much easier to do this when one is healthy. Whatever you do, if you don't have arrangements (powers of attorney,

dual signatory authority, wills, beneficiaries, etc.),
do it now! If you were sick, you wouldn't feel like
messing with it. If it were your loved one, you
wouldn't want to ask. I didn't either, but it had to be
done despite the fact that, once again, I didn't have
a clue what I was doing. There were questions to be
asked and answered.

Did Wes have a beneficiary on his accounts? I
suspected that he did on his IRA account but was
curious about his custodial account.

Wes didn't have a will, and though he'd probably been able to sign one right then, I wasn't eager
to appear to be "pushing him out the door" by
presenting him with the idea.

I hoped my broker could help. I called, and he
did.

I hoped my attorney could help. I called, and he
did.

I hoped my CPA could help. I called, and he did.

Nonetheless, I had to sit down with Wes again,
in a manner similar to what I had done before, and
ask him to sign a power of attorney to allow me
access to all his accounts so that I could handle his
affairs if his condition worsened. Again, my tears
came when I asked. He thought my requests incred-

ible and looked at me with doubt of my intentions. Wes was not happy about my asking. I believe that he read my requests as my having given up hope for him. It hurt me to hurt him in that way. I didn't see where I had a choice.

We both endured that emotional pain. Then on Monday, Claire and I had a discussion with the doctor that was more painful than anyone should have had to endure.

The blasts were above 80 percent before we started this last round. Wes was not terribly ambulatory, so he required assistance. His eyesight was failing as well. Since the last round of treatment had started, he had improved; however, the doctor didn't think the effects of the current regimen would be as effective as others had been previously. Maybe it would sustain him for a week or so. We were just trying to keep him comfortable. I hadn't told anybody, but Dr. Langston was suggesting hospice or something like it. She gave me a DNR. In case Wes had an episode at the house and was rushed to a hospital by paramedics, the DNR, or Do Not Resuscitate Order, would allow them to forgo the normal procedure of resuscitation. Claire was vehemently opposed to it, and I shared her concern. The

DNR made it seem as though we were giving up, but I realized that we needed to have the procedure in place if something were to happen. I was trying to get powers of attorney and other documents prepared without actually letting on why to Wes. I just hoped we could spare him additional pain. This was excruciatingly painful for us.

I don't know which is more painful: knowing or watching. Wes remained at home with every-other-day trips to the clinic, but his condition was not improving. Still, his spirits remained remarkable.

As you can or cannot imagine, that week was somewhat challenging. Wes's eyesight and mobility continued to deteriorate. His appetite seemed to come and go, mostly go. We made trips to the clinic on Monday, Wednesday, and Friday, and he did well the first two days. For fear of overmedicating him, I cut back on his antinausea medication on Thursday night, figuring that it had been a week since his last chemo treatment. Lo and behold, on Friday morning he awoke nauseated, and we had a terrible time getting that under control. Finally, Friday night it subsided.

The bright part of the week was Wes's friends. He'd sleep most of the day and rouse about 5:30 PM

when his friends would start coming over. He drew
such energy from them, and they were so good,
kind, and understanding. It was obvious that they
loved him, and Wes loved them so much. Different
sets of friends would come over each night, and
Wes enjoyed their visits. They visited Wes each
evening and had laughs and good times. Friday,
as he was not feeling well, the visits overwhelmed
him, and he needed some time alone. He came
to me in tears, either from his pain or the pain of
asking his friends to leave. I asked him, "Do you
want to be alone?" He said yes through his tears.
Graciously, his friends understood and left, vowing
to return when he felt better. All called the next
day, but the weather hadn't been conducive to their
return.

Claire and I attempted to rise to the challenge.
It was emotionally and physically draining, but we
drew energy from our God and our love for our son.
God blessed us with the resolve to see it through to
Wes's glory, whatever that might be. As conditions
dictated each day, we changed directions and efforts
to do what we perceived to be in Wes's overall best
interests. We believed that God was guiding us and
providing us with the strength, courage, and peace

necessary to endure those efforts, and we recognized that God was in control. He knew what must be done, and He equipped us both to meet the daily challenges we faced. We continue to be grateful for His persevering love and His strength upon which we lean for continued support.

19

The Last Dance

That Monday, we rose to take Wes to the clinic. I roused Wes to find him in more pain than normal and his eyesight and mobility further impaired. Getting him dressed and to the bathroom was a challenge and took longer than normal. When it came time to get Wes up and into the car, the walk through the kitchen proved to be extremely difficult for him, and he put more weight than normal on me for support. By the time he and I made it to the garage door and had two steps to negotiate, it was obvious that we were going to need more help. Claire, sensing our difficulties, came and took Wes under his right arm and as I was on his left, Wes let all his weight go, and Claire and I basically had to drag him to the car. Once there, though a painful exercise, Wes was glad to be able to sit. We got him situated, buckled him in, and started out to Emory. None of us said a word during the entire trip.

Once we pulled up at the front door of the clinic, I jumped out and ran around to the passenger door to help Wes disembark. During prior visits, the method I had used had been pretty successful. I would bend over at the waist, and he would lock his arms around my neck. I would stand, pulling him to an upright position. There we would stand, arm in arm, for a few moments until we were both balanced. Then, we would start the baby-step dance of turning him around to sit in the wheelchair. It was during these embraces that we would occasionally tell each other that we loved each other. The pain associated with standing was too much for such this morning.

The baby-step dance was not as choreographed as before, and when Wes went to turn, I couldn't hold his weight. He fell fairly hard into the wheelchair. He hurt, and I hurt for him. Once in the clinic, moving him from the wheelchair to the chair was another challenge. He was obviously in pain, so they administered pain medication in large doses immediately upon our arrival.

Still, Claire and I spoke little. Responding to the nurses and reacting to the needs of Wes took all we had.

Finally, the doctor came over and said, as she had a tendency to do, "How's it going?"

"Not too good today. He's in a lot of pain."

"How are you doing?" she asked to my surprise.

Without hesitation, without having to think and with complete candor, I said, "Doctor, I believe we have reached our physical limitations of being able to render effective care for Wes at home." The doctor and I both looked at Claire, and she vigorously agreed. This had not been discussed. It was simply something that we inherently knew was the right thing to do.

With that, the doctor addressed Wes, who by then had been pretty heavily medicated.

"Wes, is it a pain in the butt to come in here every day?"

Yes, he nodded.

"Would you be more comfortable in the hospital?"

Yes, he nodded.

"Well, then that's what we will do. We will discontinue the treatments as they are no longer productive. Nothing that we can do at this point can generate results that will be curative. We can, however, make you comfortable and that's what we'll do."

Shocked by the seemingly rapid turn of events, we looked up to see Claire's sister-in-law Celia standing in the clinic. She'd had an appointment of her own that morning and figuring that we might be there, came down to check.

With the curtain drawn around the cubicle, she timidly asked, "Is this a bad time? If it is, I can go . . ." With that Claire said, "No!" She grabbed her by the arm and dragged her into the cubicle with us. So in a little while, Wes was moved into a room on the sixth floor of Emory hospital.

Emory has a system of tunnels under the streets to access various buildings within the complex. The tunnels are somewhat ominous in that they echo the slightest noise and are generally inhabited by workers and patients unable to access the other areas without assistance. That morning, Wes fit into the latter category, and our nurse friend Charlotte Williams had scarcely left our side all day. When it came time to move Wes to a room in the hospital, she commandeered a wheelchair and took off into the tunnel with Wes and us in tow. As we traveled down the tunnel from the clinic to the hospital, Claire hung tight to Celia. She stayed with us the entire day and most of the night. It is times like these that reassure us how much we love and appreciate our family.

Other family had to be told. I notified Sean and Brittany. We notified my mom and Claire's parents. Word traveled fast. The stream of well-wishers, friends, and relatives started coming soon and continued late into the evening.

At one point that afternoon, once Wes was in the bed and apparently comfortable, Claire was standing at the head of the bed holding his hand, and he looked up into her face and said, "Oh, Mom, you're here." We didn't know, but we wouldn't hear from Wes again.

Late that night, after the guests had left, Wes's breathing was steady, and it appeared that, since there had been no change in his condition for hours, he would probably maintain that posture until morning, so Claire and I slipped out and drove home to catch a few hours of sleep. We were both too scared to sleep but too exhausted to stay awake. We both slept.

We arrived back at Emory on Tuesday morning to find Wes in much the same state. One of his favorite nurse techs had assured us that she would be with him all night, and she had been. Whenever her periodic rounds were completed, she sat in Wes's room and talked to him. She mentioned that Wes reminded her of her grandson.

Early that day, the parade of friends started. The most startling were the strangers. Parents of Wes's friends, most of whom we'd never met, came and gushed about what Wes meant to them and their children. Stories started coming out. Stories we'd never heard.

One father came in dressed to the nines. French cuffs and a double-breasted suit was his attire. He was an athletic looking gentleman, polished in his appearance. He asked me if I was Wes's dad and began to tell me how much he admired Wes. Then he told me that he had lost a son and that, if I ever needed anything or if I just needed to talk about the situation, he would be more than happy to meet with me. I can't begin to describe how gracious I found his visit, how generous I thought it was of him to take his time to come and counsel me.

The doctors encouraged us to continue talking to Wes, as the sense of hearing is the last thing to go. So we encouraged his friends to go in and say whatever they wanted to say, though Wes was not likely to respond. We heard the most tender and heartfelt stories, delivered passionately by these amazing young people. Many of them started with similar lines.

"Wes, you were my first friend at GACS . . ."

"Wes, you were my first friend at Georgia Perimeter College . . ."

"Wes, you were my very first friend . . ."

"Wes, you taught me that I matter . . ."

"Wes, you taught me how to love other people . . ."

And then there were the "remember when's."

These testimonies went on all afternoon and all night, with some as late as 3:00 AM.

Most had left the hospital that Tuesday night except for me, Claire, Sean, Brittany, my mother, our pastor, and one of Wes's friends. We took turns talking to Wes, holding his hand, giving him permission to go. I never thought that I could do that. I never want to do it again.

The pastor, a good friend, stayed the entire night. Not only did he not doze, I don't think he even blinked. I accused him of having learned that in seminary. They must have had a course on how to stay up all night. He finally left about 7:00 AM.

My mother also never slept. She, at eighty-nine years of age, maintained a vigil with us the entire night. Impressed by her but worried for her, I suggested that Sean take her home so that she could get some rest. They left about 8:00 AM.

Here it was Wednesday morning, and since Monday afternoon, Wes had shown little activity. He had been rhythmically breathing in what seemed to be a mildly labored fashion. It was a sight and sound that made me feel conflicted. To hear that somewhat raspy exhale let me know that he was still with us. But to hear the difficulty with which it was effected made me feel that he was struggling. Watching that effort was a difficult thing for a father to do. I questioned the doctors, and they assured us he wasn't in any discomfort. I couldn't be totally sure. The sight belied their answer.

Brittany was asleep in the chair in Wes's room, and since Wes continued to breathe his labored, rhythmic breaths, Claire and I decided to sneak

downstairs to get something to eat. Claire left Britt
a note written on a napkin that we'd gone down
to get a bite and would be right back. We weren't
really hungry but knew we needed to eat something. We went downstairs to the cafeteria and ate
our bacon and eggs very quickly. As we left the
cafeteria about ten minutes later, we ran into the
beautiful and compassionate patient coordinator
for Wes's floor, and she suggested we join her on
a different elevator than we'd used before. As we
stepped on the elevator, my cell phone rang once
and then lost signal. I figured it must have been
Brittany. In what seemed like two seconds, the
elevator door opened, and we were three steps
away from his room at the nurse's station where
we ran into Charlotte Williams, the nurse, who
was checking on Wes's condition. Claire grabbed
Charlotte by the arm and pulled her with us to the
door of Wes's room. We walked in to find Brittany
at the foot of the bed and Jessica, the PA, standing
at the head. Brittany turned to us and said, "He's
gone." It was 9:36 AM on Wednesday, February
2nd. It wasn't until that second that Claire gave up
hope for his recovery.

We all sobbed as we held hands, and I said a prayer for Wes and for us. I can't remember what I said or even how I managed to say it, but I just hope God knows and heard it.

20

Sydney's Birthday, Groundhog Day and the Trumpets

Ayoung chaplain came in and initially seemed at a loss for words. After a few minutes, he said a prayer and left. Then three of the folks from the clinic came over from across the street. I guess news travels fast in the hospital. One asked if she could pray with us. "Of course," we said, so we gathered around in a circle and held hands, and she said the most soothing words, "Father God, we know You don't make no mistakes and this ain't no mistake." I needed those words. If God was in control, then I had to trust God that Wes's death was not a mistake. The reasons for Wes's life had become much more apparent over the previous two days with the stories that had been shared by his friends, but the reason for his death had not been revealed. I simply had to trust God that it would be revealed to me in His time. I would wait.

Phone calls had to be made to the funeral home, to the grandparents, to Wes's close friends, and they were asked to notify others. When asked by hospital personnel our preference of funeral homes, I had them contact the family funeral home that had taken care of my dad twenty-two years earlier on February 13, 1982. Once they had come to the hospital and collected the precious cargo, Claire and I prepared to head home. While I'd gone to get the car, Claire and Charlotte remained in the room. Charlotte turned to Claire and said, "This is the last time you'll be in this room. Is there anything that you want?" Claire replied, "I want his pillowcase." With that, Charlotte ripped the pillowcase off the pillow where Wes's head had gone to eternal rest. She folded the linen and pressed it against Claire's cheek. Claire breathed in all of Wes that remained in the fabric of that case and the fabric absorbed her tears.

We rode home in a daze. I don't recall saying a word.

Upon arriving home, we found that Claire's brother and nephew, Robert and Josh, were there and Robert was answering the phone and taking messages. I went to my office to formulate a funeral notice and put out the following e-mail.

It is with extreme grief and celebration that I announce that at 9:31 AM on February 2, 2005, the trumpets of heaven heralded Wes's entrance into the arms of Jesus. Your persistent prayers on Wes's behalf are no longer necessary as he is in the loving care of the One to whom we pray. Wes would want you to know how much he appreciated and was awed by your love and prayerfulness. Though he could not personally thank each of you, he constantly relayed to Claire and me how much your prayers meant to him. He was blessed by your constant love.

Claire and I thank God for lending us His child. Our prayer upon Wes's passing was of thanksgiving for Wes's life, his spirit, his wisdom beyond his years, the lessons he

taught his parents, and the love he shared
with all his friends and family. We can brag
on him a little since he was God's child first.
He was remarkable.

His parents are going to need some time
to compose and grieve. Second Samuel
12:15–23 states:

Then Nathan went to his house. The LORD
struck the child that Uriah's wife bore to
David, and it became very ill. David therefore pleaded with God for the child; David
fasted, and went in and lay all night on the
ground. The elders of his house stood beside
him, urging him to rise from the ground; but
he would not, nor did he eat food with them.
On the seventh day the child died. And the
servants of David were afraid to tell him that
the child was dead; for they said, "While the
child was still alive, we spoke to him, and
he did not listen to us; how then can we tell
him the child is dead? He may do himself
some harm." But when David saw that
his servants were whispering together, he
perceived that the child was dead; and David

said to his servants, "Is the child dead?"
They said, "He is dead." Then David rose
from the ground, washed, anointed himself,
and changed his clothes. He went into the
house of the LORD, and worshiped; he then
went to his own house; and when he asked,
they set food before him and he ate. Then
his servants said to him, "What is this thing
that you have done? You fasted and wept for
the child while it was alive; but when the
child died, you rose and ate food." He said,
"While the child was still alive, I fasted and
wept; for I said, 'Who knows? The LORD
may be gracious to me, and the child may
live.' But now he is dead; why should I fast?
Can I bring him back again? I shall go to
him, but he will not return to me."

Wes is in a good place, free from pain,
free from chemo, free from needles, free
from infusions. Why would he choose to
come back here? He wouldn't. So we'll go
to him. Not today but soon in relation to the
eternity we'll spend together.

We pray for the Lord's strength, courage, and power that He provided David upon his loss.

Praise God for the life of Wes.

Funeral arrangements will follow later as completed.

WES

While I was doing that, Claire approached Josh and said, "I don't think I can do this, Josh." Josh said, "Yes you can, Aunt Claire." But Claire persisted, "No, Josh, you know how, when someone gets married, there's a wedding coordinator? I need a funeral coordinator. Are there those kinds of people?" "I don't think so," was his answer.

At that very second, the back door opened and in walked five of Claire's Bible study members from our community. Stephanie walked directly up to Claire, hugged her, offered her condolences, and said, "Okay, here's what you're going to do. You and Smitty are going to go lie down and get a few hours of sleep. When you wake up, you need to get a shower and get dressed and come back in here because this place is going to be full of people. Don't worry about anything. Do not answer the phone. Everything will be handled by us. This area is off limits. You are to do nothing. Now go!"

The funeral coordinator had arrived.

And they did exactly that. They took care of everything. Someone was assigned to answer the telephone. A book was placed next to it to log the calls with who called, when, and about what. There was another logbook to list who brought food and another for who sent flowers. Each day, they let us sleep and have a little quiet time in the morning and would come to the house at about 10:00 AM and stay until 10:00 or 11:00 PM. We were at their mercy and glad for it.

One bit of advice that would have slipped past us was the advice to stay hydrated. We were encouraged to keep water with us at all times and drink it constantly. Crying and the sniffles that go along with it deplete your body of water. Rehydrating was necessary to maintain our strength for all that was to go on.

Uncharacteristically, I didn't want to drive anywhere. Claire's brother Robert acted as our chauffeur. If something needed to be done, I simply told Robert, and he would handle it. What a blessing. I was in such a poor mental state; I surrendered to those who asked to help.

On Thursday afternoon we had to meet with the funeral home and take Wes's burial clothes and attend to the plans. To our delight the folks at the funeral home were professionals in all respects. They were compassionate, caring, calming, and attentive. They anticipated our needs and responded in a timely fashion. They approached Wes's service with dignity and pride and saw to the pertinence of each detail.

In Wes's later years, though he'd been voted best dressed in high school for his choice of suits and general demeanor, he'd taken a more casual approach to attire. Jeans replaced slacks. Sweaters or sweatshirts replaced sport coats. And since his hair had fallen out and he'd received repeated sunburns on his pate, a stocking cap with a small brim had personified Wes. To that end, Wes would not have looked right in a suit. So Wes was buried in his designer jeans, his designer tennis shoes, his trademark Honda T-shirt, a tan wool sweater that he loved to wear, and his stocking cap. During the viewing, we included his watch, his Live Strong bracelet, his rings, and his signature sunglasses perched on his forehead. He looked peaceful.

Upon arriving home that afternoon, we walked in the house to find my office phone receiving the last of a voice mail from Tom Reynolds. Tom was a dealer friend of mine I'd been acquainted with but not really known. Claire and I had found out late last year that Tom's wife, Pat, was suffering from two types of cancer and was being treated at Emory. Our paths crossed often during Wes's and Pat's treatments.

Though Tom and I had a friendship, he and Claire forged a bond one Sunday when both Wes and Pat were in the clinic for treatments. On those days the clinic was basically closed. Only a skeleton crew was at work to attend to emergency needs of patients who needed platelets or blood infusions.

While both of the patients were receiving treatments with uneventful results, Tom and Claire found themselves at the main desk. After making a little small talk, Tom asked if he could buy Claire a cup of coffee. The coffee was free. Claire knew that, but it was still sweet of Tom to ask, and so Claire smiled and accepted his offer.

Coffee poured, Tom opened with some heartfelt comments about how he was feeling. He was scared and depressed about his wife's condition. He went

on to confide that he had previously experienced
a heart condition and, during that time, had been
terribly depressed and continued to fight that demon
when faced with Pat's prognosis. Who wouldn't?

Claire seized the opportunity to tell her story.
You see, while Claire was undergoing chemotherapy for breast cancer, there was one day when
she rose with certain things to do. That morning,
after finally mustering the strength to take a bath,
she sat in the garden tub of our home in Stone
Mountain, stared at her bald self in the mirror, and
held a pity party. She started to talk to God.

"Okay, God, what's going on? Is this just some
sort of cruel joke? Are You making me go through
all this just to die anyway?"

To her dismay, the mirrors didn't crack, and God
didn't appear with the cure in His hands. She did,
however, have a thought that resounded in her head.

"Oh, you of little faith . . ." (Matthew 6:30 NIV).

"But, God, I feel so bad. I ache. I don't have any
energy. This is unfair! Are You just kidding me?"

"Oh, you of little faith . . ." (Matthew 6:30 NIV).

"Okay, Lord. I've got three things that I need
to do today. Just three, but I need Your help. I need
to get dressed, I need to vacuum the house, and I

need to bake some chocolate-chip cookies for Sean because he's coming home from school today. Please, Lord, just give me the strength to do those three things."

Once out of the tub, dressed, and attempting to put on some makeup, Claire heard a noise emanating from upstairs. This noise had never been heard unless Claire was responsible for it. After some confusion, she recognized the sound of a vacuum cleaner. Brittany, who heretofore had been unaware of what a vacuum cleaner was or how it worked, was—without provocation, request, or even suggestion—vacuuming the upstairs.

Then the telephone rang. Claire, already tired, decided to allow the answering machine to pick up.

After a few rings, it stopped.

A few minutes later, Britt came downstairs and started talking.

"Mom, Jeannie called and said . . ."

Claire cut her off in mid sentence. "Just tell her that I don't feel up to it today and to call me again some other time."

Now it was Britt's turn to cut Claire off. "Mom, it's too late. She's already hung up, and she's on the way over."

Despondent over the news, Claire continued getting ready and prepared to meet her guest. In just a matter of minutes, there was a knock on the door.

Jeannie is a wonderful lady with a sweet smile, a peaceful countenance, and a bubbly personality. True to form, she came in the door talking.

"Hi, Claire, I hope you're feeling okay this morning. Look, last night was Tom's company Christmas party. We had it at the house and wouldn't you know it, I've been cooking and baking all week. I get all this stuff made, and they come and don't eat it all, so we've got tons of stuff left over."

Then, from behind her back, Jeannie pulled out a huge bag of chocolate chip cookies, without nuts, important only because Sean hates nuts.

"So I brought these to you . . ."

Claire was stunned.

Then Jeannie, not realizing the prayer request she had just filled, continued talking, "Oh, wait a minute, I almost forgot, I've got to get your present out of my car." She quickly disappeared out the door.

In a few seconds she reappeared, ushered Claire into the den, sat her down, and insisted she open her present right then. Claire complied and found in the box a stuffed bear. Now Claire was a bear collector at the time, but this bear had special significance. It was wearing a little Santa hat, but more importantly, it held a stocking that had emblazoned on its cuff, the word "Believe."

"Oh, you of little faith . . . believe."

Right there, on that morning, in that place, Claire knew for certain that God loves her and does answer prayers. She'd asked for three things and all three were accomplished in less than an hour. She also knew that God was not playing games but had plans for her beyond breast cancer.

And so it was with the story that Claire imparted to Tom. Just believe. If God could answer her three needs on one morning so obviously and so completely, He could handle Tom's. According to Tom, that assurance helped him through many difficult times.

This day, however, the ringing phone was Tom calling to leave a message to tell me that Pat had passed away on Tuesday evening. I immediately picked up the phone and called Tom to give him my condolences and to tell him about Wes. He and Pat were in heaven together. What a coincidence.

Ironically, the year Wes was born, the same
family funeral home that was attending to Wes was
asked to bury my dad. They had been exemplary
in their work and had even called me back to the
funeral home after the interment to say that, when
lowering my dad's casket into the grave, a belt had
slipped, the casket slid against some equipment and
had been damaged, and they had brought him back
and replaced the damaged casket. They asked if I
would come back and satisfy myself that my dad
and his accommodations were satisfactory. I went.
They were, and I thought that their call was an indication of their integrity, so when it came time to
call someone for Wes, they were the natural choice.
They did not disappoint me.

The viewing for Wes was Friday night. It started
at 6:00 PM and was to conclude at 8:30 PM. People
arrived at 5:45 PM, and the first people Claire and I
saw were two folks we didn't know very well but
who had recently joined our Sunday-school class.
As we walked in, we found Joel and Susan Gilbert
carefully studying a couple of bulletin boards of
photos the funeral home had placed on easels in
the viewing room. The photos were of Wes and his
friends. Joel approached me after what seemed like

a very long time looking at the boards and said, "I never had an opportunity to meet Wes, but after having heard you speak of him and studying these pictures, I believe I have a sense of who he was. That is my loss. I think I would have liked him." I'm sure Wes would have liked Joel too.

Within what seemed like minutes of our arrival, a line formed that led out the door and around the outside of the building. Claire and I, initially together to greet people, got separated and two lines were formed to speed up the flow. Some people waited more than an hour in line. Wes had so many friends. Some traveled from as far away as Oregon, Mississippi, and Missouri. Our church friends and my previous employees graciously came to show their respects to us and to Wes. We continued to be awed by the love of God that was exhibited through all those people.

As the night wound to a close about 9:30 PM, the family gathered around the casket to say goodnight to Wes, and Claire said, "We'll see you tomorrow, baby." At that point, I had to say, "No, darling, you won't. If we have good-byes to say, we need to say them tonight because the coffin won't be open tomorrow." "Why?" she persisted. "Hon, they just

don't do that. The closing of the casket is too traumatic in and of itself. If it were done just before
the funeral, you couldn't regain your composure to
receive any benefit from the service." She conceded.
She, Brittany, Sean, and I said our good-byes, and
then, as the most natural thing I've ever done, I asked
them all to pray with me. I reached down, grabbed
Wes's hands, and recited, to the best of my recollection the blessing from the book of Numbers 6:24–26:

> *Now may the Lord bless you and keep you.*
> *May the Lord make His face to shine upon*
>   *you and be gracious unto you.*
> *May the Lord grant you His peace both now*
>   *and forever more.*
> *Amen*

That was the last time any of us saw Wes—for
now.

Again, we returned home, and this night there
were very few people. The number was just enough
to see that we were fed and settled and ready to
retire. Arrangements were made for the next day, for
gathering all the folks who needed to be gathered
and shuttled to the funeral.

21

Helping Billy Cry

We rose the following morning to a beautiful day. For Wes it was a day he would have ordered. Clearly, it was a top-down day. It could not have been more perfect.

That morning, family gathered at the house and Claire, Sean, Britt, my mother, Claire's mom and dad, my brother's wife, Carol, his daughter Catherine, Claire's best friend from North Carolina, Cindy, and I piled into the limousines sent over by the funeral home and made the twenty-one-mile trek from Duluth to Smoke Rise Baptist Church in Stone Mountain.

We had started attending Smoke Rise Baptist Church before Wes was born. He was baptized there. Needless to say, we were all grief stricken, devastated, and emotionally spent, but when we reached the back doors of the sanctuary to file in as a family, as the doors opened and revealed the white woodwork, white pews, and burgundy carpet I had seen so many times before, there was an energy that flowed from within that seemed uncommon. And then, the source of that energy became apparent. I had never seen so many people in that church in my life. Every pew was filled, even in the balcony. I struggled to hold back the tears because all those people were there for either Wes or us. How kind. How generous of their time to give up their day to pay tribute to the Smiths. I was humbled.

Music was an important part of Wes's life, and so it had to be an important part of his service. Whatever music was played had to have relevance. It, too, had to tell a story. After the congregation was seated and the ministers had prayer with the family, we were led into the instrumental version of "A Mighty Fortress Is Our God." How true those words were. Without the strength and fortress provided by our God, we would not have had the strength or courage to face that day.

Wes's service began and, like the day, was beautiful and a wonderful tribute to a special young man. I think Wes would have been proud.

One of Wes's friends from Savannah had agreed to perform the song by Mercy Me, "I Can Only Imagine." Wes loved the song and sang it often. It could have been because he was planning what he would do when he met Jesus. I had never heard Scotty sing or play the guitar, but Wes had spoken often about Scotty's talent. Wes was a huge Scotty fan. Unheard, I trusted Wes's judgment. Scotty nailed it! I was so proud of him, and I knew Wes was too.

The most amazing thing happened within the first day or so of Wes's death. Jessica Neely, one of the physician's assistants who had been attending to Wes throughout his treatment, asked a dear friend of ours if we might let her speak at Wes's ceremony. Delighted that she would make such a generous offer, we accepted. As she was preparing her remarks, she asked Wes's oncologist, Dr. Winton, for some suggestions of what she should say. To our surprise, he asked her, "Do you think they would let me speak too?"

I understand that it is highly unusual for attending physicians to speak at funerals. But, of course, we learned that things that might be unusual for some folks didn't seem that unusual where Wes was concerned.

Both spoke of Wes's courage and strength, of his spirit and his humor. They spoke of his giving nature and his cooperative initiative to help and encourage other patients. They both spoke of their dedication to find a cure for the leukemia that took Wes, and both spoke of the love they had developed for him.

Dr. Truett Gannon, our minister for many years, graciously spoke too. As always, his message was calm, kind, to the point, and uplifting. One comment he made touched many. He said, "Children can never love parents as much as the parent can love the child." Never having truly thought about it, I now believe it to be true. But he went on to say that "for God, death is the moment when one of His children comes home."

Dr. Gannon went on to compare Wes's last year with the five most difficult years during World War II that Winston Churchill ascribed as England's finest hour. Wes's last year was such a contrast to his first twenty-one. It was so uncharacteristically difficult, yet Wes held his head high and persevered through every single day. Dr. Gannon said it was his finest hour because "trauma doesn't make character as much as it reveals character."

We will be forever indebted to Dr. Gannon for his love, counsel, and friendship. He has been omnipresent in our lives during difficult times and always had the right words to give us comfort. Wes's ceremony was no exception.

Two of Wes's friends spoke of the type of friend Wes was. They spoke of how he thought of others first and how he just wanted to "be." If he was with them, he was fine. He didn't need a lot to entertain him; he just wanted his friends close. That was enough.

To his tribute, Sean spoke. I don't know how he did it, but he spoke with grace and dignity and eloquence. Words are inadequate to express how proud it makes a father to have one son speak so reverently of another son in such a public arena. Sean spoke of how Wes professed his love for him when he was in the deepest pain he had experienced. Through his pain, Wes thought of his brother. Sean, trying desperately to comfort Wes, was trying to find out what he could do to help ease his pain. "What do you want me to do, Wes?" Then, barely able to speak, Wes looked at Sean and simply said, "I sure do love you." Watching Wes in pain was originally the last place Sean wanted to be but receiving the blessing from Wes transformed it into the only place he wanted to be.

Lastly, our youth minister, Ernie Forrester, delivered the eulogy. Rarely at a loss for words and always with a casual, comfortable, and sincere delivery, Ernie remained true to form. He told some funny stories about what Wes did when he was at the church and how Wes seemed to keep Ernie hopping because Ernie never knew what to expect from Wes. But whatever it was, it would be fun.

Ernie contrasted Wes's fun-loving demeanor with a visit to the hospital in the summer. Claire and I had gone to get something to eat, and Wes got serious with Ernie. He told him his greatest fear. It wasn't of death. Ernie said that Wes shared that he was ready. His fear, as was customary of Wes, involved thinking of others. He feared that some of his friends would not meet him in heaven because they had not accepted Christ. "I just don't know if they all know." Later, you'll see why Wes's fear, his expression of it, and the importance of Ernie's message continues to keep Wes's spirit alive.

Ernie closed with the following comment, "The demon that is leukemia has taken Wes's body, but the demon that is leukemia could never take away Wes's spirit or the memory we have of him."

A friend of Brittany's that had become just as good a friend to Wes spoke at the service, and I had asked her to sing "Because He Lives." Pertinent again to the moment, we collectively knew that the only way we could face the next day after our devastating loss was through the grace of God. Because Christ lives in us, we can do all things, even if it includes going on after burying a child.

Dr. Browning, our pastor, then closed the ceremony with these words, "May the God who has laughed and cried with us today go with us, granting us the strength that we need to face our tomorrows to continue Wes's good work, to heal our hearts. Amen."

With that we rose, and, as a family, started to file out the side door of the sanctuary. Many of our friends, some we had not seen in years, lined the sidewalk between the door and the limo. Able only to speak briefly to a soccer coach of Wes's from when he was about nine years old (How did he know?) and only able to acknowledge some of the nurses from the hospital, we filed into the limo.

Settled in and sitting between Claire and my
mother, still reeling from the service, I looked
out and saw our dear friend Tom standing on the
sidewalk.

What a tribute to us and Wes for Tom to come to
Wes's celebration with his wife's passing so fresh. I
had to get to him.

I imposed on my mom to get out just so that
I could find Tom and throw my arms around him.
I did so with great appreciation for his unselfish
gesture. It spoke volumes of his character. Tom is a
godly man.

While we were still numb with shock and I was
once again back inside the limo, the driver pulled
out to follow Wes's hearse and lead the processional
to the cemetery. But through that numbness, one
vision touched me deeply. As we took a right turn
out of the church parking lot, moving at a crawl,
I looked to my right and saw the father of one of
Wes's friends standing next to his car at military
attention saluting the processional. This was a
friend that Wes had tried desperately to help find the
right side of the path of life, to no avail. The father's
gesture was one of kindness and respect and one
that will never be forgotten.

Once we arrived at the gravesite, I was amazed to see how many people had come from the church service because the cemetery is about fifteen or more miles from the church. I had expected a handful, but there were at least a hundred.

The sight of Wes's friends acting as pallbearers caused my eyes to well up with tears. Jared, Richard, Brandon, Ryan, Trey, Shane, Noah, and Brad were young men shouldering the burden of Wes's casket and the burden of their own loss. Some had never been in a suit before, but in honor of Wes they dressed up this day. They all looked so distinguished and made me very proud.

My eyes welled up again when, after the casket was lowered, one by one, they each threw their red rose boutonniere into the grave on top of the casket. What a tribute from some classy young men.

Fortunately, God took over for me because I was too numb and emotional to speak on my own. As the pastors finished their presentations and prayers, from somewhere deep inside me, God provided these words: "Thank you for coming to honor our son. As Wes always drew strength and comfort from his friends, at this time, we will seek to do the same."

We visited on that cemetery hillside with many friends, relatives, and many strangers who came to pay their respects. Some appeared more emotional than we were, though my guess would be that we were simply numb.

I don't know how long we stayed there at the cemetery. At some point, it was determined that it was time to go, though neither Claire nor I wanted to leave. It didn't seem right to leave Wes there on that hill. Yet, we left.

Unbeknownst to us, the funeral coordinators were having some difficulties back at the house. A local social club had been advised of our loss and offered to prepare food for the family for Saturday afternoon. It was a kind and generous offer. Someone was to arrive at the club at about 1:00 PM on Saturday and simply pick up the food. On Saturday the designated "someone" arrived at the club only to find it closed and locked. The club, for whatever reason, did not fulfill that commitment. When the funeral coordinator heard this news, she went into immediate despair.

"What will we do? We have hundreds of people on the way over, and they'll be hungry. Oh, God, what shall we do?"

Not minutes later, but that very second, the doorbell rang. When answered, there stood someone from our Sunday-school class asking, "What do you want me to do with all this food? I've got two trucks full and just need to know where you want me to put it."

Like the fishes and loaves, God had seen, once again, that the multitudes would be fed and fed in abundance.

Upon arriving home, it was apparent that our funeral coordinators were busy rushing around in the kitchen with their matching blue aprons seeing to it that everyone was fed and "watered." Before we could make it from the front door to the kitchen, a glass of white wine was handed to Claire and my favorite drink was handed to me. There was food everywhere, so we knew nothing of the earlier food supply problem until much later. Fortunately, the gloom that had hung over the house that day was replaced with stories of Wes and laughter of his antics. The house was abuzz. Familiar faces, equally strange faces, aromas of food, and sounds of people paying tribute to our son and us were everywhere. It was quite a comfort to have them here, but when the night wore down and all the guests had trickled out and the loneliness of home began to creep back in like a fog, there was a void that we will never be able to fill.

We received a kind e-mail from a friend who had lost a daughter years earlier. She was one of those who "knew." Yet, her grace and kindness showed in her heartfelt words and helped to soothe us. If she said it, it must be true because she "knew."

Dear Bill and Claire,

The service for Wes was perfect. What a lovely tribute to him. Just think of all the people who were inspired that day! Even the weather reflected the mood—the sun was shining so brightly and it truly was a celebration! Sean did a wonderful job, and I was so proud of him. Those five words will be with him forever. I always told my children that the best thing in life is shared moments with family and friends—some funny, silly, or touching, but those are the things we hold dear in our hearts always.

You and Claire are just awesome, and I am so happy to know you.

I have fond memories of Wes, and
they'll always be in my heart.

We attended church the morning following the
funeral. It was just something we needed to do. It
was extremely painful, and we did our best to hold it
together. Sometimes we did. Sometimes we didn't.
The sanctuary that had housed so many of Wes's
friends the day before felt quite different on the
following day. It felt cavernous and somewhat eerie.
The previous day, it had felt cozy and warm. The
spirit of the moment must define the space, wherever
and whatever that place may be. We did pretty well
throughout Sunday school and the service until the
choir sang "the prayer," the verses from Numbers
that I had spoken to Wes the night before his funeral,
as the benediction. We both lost it.

But one couple happened to see us there and
wrote us an account of how they felt.

I guess we will all understand things much
better in heaven or maybe there will be no
need, but it sure is hard to understand why
such good people have to endure such great
sufferings on this earth, WES. No one knows

how they will handle things until they are put into a situation . . . I have learned that in my fifty-seven years of living. You have handled your situations so beautifully and with such grace. I saw you and Claire come into church Sunday. You know, I think that when I see you, I just see faith walking. You both have become our examples. I hope that doesn't make you uncomfortable. And you are entitled to feel whatever you feel with all that you have been through and continue to experience. But no matter what, the journey you have walked and shared will have forever changed many of our lives, and we thank you for making us better people. Keep up the journaling if it helps you. It sure is a blessing to us.

Once again, we were labeled as "examples." Many times, people said we were "an inspiration." Don't misunderstand; I appreciated their generous words, but to be candid I didn't set out to be an example, and if I'd had a choice, which I didn't, of being an inspiration or having my son back, I'd take my boy, hands down. Losing him just hurt so much. Yet we had to endure and persevere.

We went through the motions one goes through when a loss occurs in the family. Most of the time, we were lucky to get our feet under us to stand. Actually, we felt lost. During the year that Wes was in the hospital, every minute of our days was consumed with him or his treatment. Between his death and the funeral, each day was consumed with arrangements. Now, we had to make a conscious decision about what we would do each day. The exercise seemed foreign. Each day showed some improvement.

When I rose the following Wednesday, I was struck rather abruptly with the realization that it had been exactly one week. It seemed much closer. As well, I knew an obligation loomed, and I didn't want to do it. After all, it was Claire's birthday, and I couldn't imagine anyone, especially her, especially after what we'd been through, wanting to spend her birthday going to a funeral. But we did and, surprisingly, it felt pretty good.

For our friend Tom and for ourselves, we attended Pat's memorial service. Much like Wes's, it was a celebration and much to our surprise, we came out feeling uplifted by the service and speakers. Their son spoke and related a story I find pertinent, and I'd like to borrow it to apply it to those friends who supported us through our ordeal.

> Little Johnny was late returning from school one day, and his mother questioned why he was late.
>
> Johnny said, "Billy's bike had broken, and I stopped to help."
>
> "Johnny," Mom said, "you don't know how to fix bikes."
>
> To which Johnny replied, "I know, Mom; I didn't stop to fix the bike. I stopped to help Billy cry."

Well, that's what those friends did for us with their attendance at the visitation, the celebration, the cards, the e-mails, the visits, and the host of other kindnesses that had been shown to us. They helped us cry. They helped Billy and Claire cry. Like Johnny, they couldn't fix the problem, but they could sure help us cry. And that, my friends, was more than enough.

The funeral for Pat was cathartic. It was a celebration of her life as much as we tried to make Wes's a celebration of his. Her son spoke fondly and humorously about his mother. How he managed to do that at such a time, I'll never know.

Some of the music we had chosen for Wes's service had been chosen for Pat's. Hearing it again that day, so soon, had the effect of allowing us two services to recognize our sweet son's passing. Then, at the end of the service, the benediction was the blessing from Numbers. We simply found holding back the tears too huge a task. Again, we lost it.

We hadn't heard that benediction in years and then all of a sudden, it haunted us. It's probably just Wes saying, "I heard you, Dad." We can hope.

22

Feedback and the Confession

Writing the e-mails week after week had, indeed, been a mixed bag. It was torturous to relive the weeks but cathartic to express my feelings and especially uplifting to receive the occasional cryptic e-mail, "We are praying for you." I was going to miss the venue that the e-mails provided to vent, but I had been encouraged by many to continue.

Here are a few of the e-mails I received that were especially uplifting. It's mind-boggling to think how pervasive e-mails really are, but we were reminded of it often.

I just want you to know that there are people whom you don't know who are praying for you. I pray that God will bring His comfort and continual blessings to you.
Scott

I didn't know Scott. I still don't, but I appreciated his prayers.

Jim and I truly are amazed at both of you and your constant faith. We have prayed for your family and have asked for prayer for you, Wes, and your family from many other friends. You have truly witnessed God's love through all of this. We can only think of how it is to lose a child . . . but more importantly how you have witnessed to all of us who have not lost one. Thank you . . . for opening yourself up and letting everyone know about your feelings and pain. . . . We miss Wes . . . but mostly . . . we love your family and pray that the healing has begun.

I really wish we hadn't had to be witnesses to this part of our life. But there probably was a reason why we were.

Bill, if you can continue to muster up these e-mails, I think it's awesome! There are many of us who want to continue to support, love, and pray for your family and don't know how. But most importantly, you are an incredible witness to many. Some of whom may just need to understand what a REAL father is, but also, many others who will deal with future losses too. You are so much on track, and it's such an honor to be called your friend. Wes is SO PROUD of you too!

People continued to write similar words of encouragement over and over. It was as if they were deriving some benefit from hearing the story we had to tell. It was a new situation for me in the beginning, and it was no more comfortable after Wes's passing.

Some who received the original posts acted as switchboard operators, resending the e-mails to others in their address books. They, in turn, would receive replies and accumulate them and then forward them to me embedded in their own e-mails.

Hi, Bill and Claire,

You both continue to be in my prayers. Your willingness to share your pain and grief in your letters in order to help others is so very uplifting. As a hospice volunteer and grief support group helper, I appreciate all you have to teach me so that I may help those who are experiencing the loss of a loved one. You just don't know how much YOUR ministry has the potential to help many others. I do appreciate it, and I grieve the loss of Wes with you all.

I share your updates with the Sunday school class and I asked them today, as I sent your update, if they wished to continue getting them. Here are a few of the responses I got that I'm sure they won't mind if I share. Some know you personally and some don't, but now feel they do through your writings . . . All of them have prayed for you through this!

They are amazing to read. It's like looking deep inside someone's heart.

I love them and they bless me so. Thanks for them.

Marcia, please keep sending the updates for me. It is such a powerful testimony.

I would certainly appreciate being included in the correspondence from the Smiths. Please keep me on the list. Bill has such a gift for expressing the features of their journey, and he is so generous in sharing it; I need to be enriched by his words and thoughts. I doubt he has any idea how many folks he is touching with this part of his ministry.

I enjoy reading them. Bill has a real gift for writing. He is really

putting together something that I
believe could be published, though
he probably wouldn't want that . . .

You are blessed and you in turn are
blessing others. Thank you, Bill.

It was humbling to read those kind words. Yet, I still couldn't get over the fact that anyone could find what I had to say interesting. I felt like I had somehow been impertinent in using people's in-boxes to vent.

I had been asked by many to continue the e-mail updates. At first, I was reluctant. Then I came to the realization that walking through the grief process with Claire and me might help someone else. I asked the recipients to tell me if they were not among those "someone's" so that I could take their names off the list. As always, I didn't wish to be an unwelcome guest in anyone's in-box.

Sitting down each week during the past year to provide e-mail updates was a torturous task. It forced me to come to grips with my thoughts. Often, as I sat down, my emotions were conflicted. I realized that I could not be uncertain. Those that wanted to know wouldn't tolerate that. I could be wrong, but never uncertain. So, as I sat down to write, it was necessary to reconcile my emotions and, often, I would pray that God would grant me that peace that surpasses all understanding. In that receipt came clarity of my feelings. Then and only then could I write.

In those very seconds and in large degree today, I find myself in much the same situation. I was and remain conflicted.

Wes is with God. I know that and that is good.

Wes is missing from our home, irrespective of his condition, and that hurts deeply. It has since the day he went to be with the Lord.

We hurt tonight. We'll hurt tomorrow. Claire and I deal with this differently. I can't go in his room. She feels close to him there.

Wes was a generous soul. He'd give away his lunch money to a kid who forgot his. Charity was his thing. We'd spent most of the first week trying to be like Wes. We made donations that he would have made in honor of some people that he loved immensely.

We had to force ourselves to read the sympathy cards we received. We'd cry at the sentiment expressed, sometimes by total strangers. God's love is present in so many people. His love is abundant.

Anytime one goes through a traumatic experience, he or she is forced to deal with new "firsts": the first time at the laundry, the first time at the pharmacy, the first time at the grocery. So on and so on. If those there don't know, they ask, and you have to tell them that Wes is gone. If they do know, they express their condolences and you have to try to bear up underneath it all.

Anything could set us off and did.

During those times, our emotions were sensitized to a point that they felt that they were on our sleeves. We'd be doing fine one minute and the next . . . BAM. It was like a frying pan had hit us between the eyes. Fortunately, Claire and I were together. We'd cry together. We'd recover together.

Our prayer each night was for the courage and strength necessary to face another day and another week without our young son. It was for the strength and courage for our other children to help them deal with the loss and to use the occasion to draw them closer to each other and to us. And it was to thank God for loving us and getting us that far.

We knew that our friends and family had been praying for us. Their support and generous spirits bolstered our strength and allowed us to face each new day with hope that we would all be reunited in the blink of an eye.

This love we had been receiving from so many for so long drew us closer to our friends. When life seemed the bleakest, we'd receive a card, a phone call, or an e-mail from someone that just said simply, "We love you." Those three words provided the props to hold us up when our own strength was inadequate.

The bonds created by those words had given new meaning to our life. Because of that bond, it was with some great distress that I felt compelled to confess something that, up to this point, I had been withholding from them. And I've been withholding it from you too.

> "Everything is permissible"—but not every-thing is beneficial. "Everything is permis-sible"—but not everything is constructive. Nobody should seek his own good, but the good of others.
>
> (1 Corinthians 10:23–24 NIV)

I guess, to some degree, every relationship has boundaries. Though our friends' love and concern and diligent prayerfulness for us had appeared boundless, and despite our overwhelming gratitude for their affection, I must confess, I wasn't completely candid during Wes's illness. Allow me to explain.

Back in October of last year, Wes, Claire, and I were at the clinic receiving Wes's treatment and the doctor called and asked me to step to her office. I did. She asked, "How's it going?" I started rattling off Wes's response to medication, etc., and I realized that she was not interested in that. "I don't know doctor," I said. "How *is* it going?" She shook her head with an expression that let me know that Emory was at the end of their professional rope. "How long has he got?" I inquired.

"Two weeks to two months, depending on how comfortable we can keep him." I must have appeared catatonic because the next thing I heard was, "What do you want us to do?"

My response startled her.

"Doctor, no parent on this earth should ever have to answer that question once much less twice."

Flashback

July 30, 1985, at about 4:00 PM, I was called to my home from work due to an emergency situation involving Claire who had been relegated to bed rest since April with an uncooperative pregnancy. When I got there, the paramedics were taking my newborn daughter, Megan, out the front window of the bedroom wrapped in an aluminum foil blanket while other EMTs administered to Claire, checking off what I gathered to be very weak vital signs. Upon Claire's stabilization, they took her to one hospital and took Megan to another. My mother was with Sean and Britt, Claire's mom was with her, so that left me to go to the other hospital to attend to Megan.

Quite a while later (I don't know how long but it must have been hours because it was dark outside, in July, with daylight savings time during which time I had been praying with all my might) a doctor came outside and asked me, "Are you the father?"

I replied affirmatively, and he started in: "There has been no viable recorded birth with a gram weight less than . . ."

I interrupted, "Doctor, don't talk to me about gram weight. Talk to me about vital signs, blood pressure, heartbeat, respiration, etc."

He implored, "What do you want us to do?

"What I want you to do, doctor, is go back in there and get the top neonatal specialists you can find on the phone and find out how to save my daughter."

He revolved on his paper shoes and disappeared for what seemed like another hour. Upon the doctor's return, having been sufficiently satisfied with his response and with the names and recorded efforts he had made in trying to establish some hope for my young daughter's viability, I heard him ask once again, "What do you want us to do?"

"Doctor, do what you must."

Flash Forward

Nineteen years later, I have agonized and questioned my previous reaction to that same question countless times. Did I do all that I could do for Megan? Was there anyone, anywhere who had anything that could have changed that outcome?

Had I been unfaithful to God for not having done more? Why? Why me? Why now? Why again?

I had asked the doctor to explore all known clinical trials to see if Wes could be considered for them. I'd done Internet research to see if I could find conventional or unconventional medicine or treatments for his survival. I'd called the Fred Hutchinson Cancer Clinic in Seattle and spoken with a bone marrow transplant specialist. I wanted to be sure that I had taken whatever extra steps I may not have taken with Megan.

It was at this time that I, a previously self-employed entrepreneur who was used to attempting to control everything within my path, came to the realization that this situation was out of my control. There was nothing I could do to change the outcome of Wes's illness any more than I could have changed the outcome of Megan's life. Here was where I found the difference between *faith* and *trust*. The step in between was *surrender*. Like Abraham and Isaac, I had to completely surrender Wes to God. Total loss of control. Total reliance on God and His will, whatever it might be. It is a bit ironic that in the Scriptures the surrender of Isaac to God was for the sake of proving Abraham's obedience, trust, and faithfulness; in the surrender of Isaac, God got Abraham. So, I believe, it was in my surrender of Wes. When I surrendered Wes, my relationship with God changed. I still didn't know God's will for Wes, but I knew that whatever it was, it would be okay.

We all continued to pray for a miracle for Wes. We knew then and know now that God is the Great Physician. If it were His will to heal Wes, it could have and would have been done. I couldn't tell Claire what the doctor had told me. It would have destroyed her hope. Likewise, I was afraid to tell our friends for fear that they, too, would give up hope. I couldn't tell Wes what the doctor said because I wanted him in the right frame of mind to receive God's miracle if God chose to bestow it upon him. But, as it played out, I realized even more that I was praying for my miracle, Claire was praying for her miracle, and neither of those was Wes's miracle. That wasn't a mistake. God doesn't make mistakes. That was where Wes was destined to be. And it is where we too will be in our time.

I hope you will accept my apology for withholding information until now. I just didn't know what to do. I didn't know how to tell you in fear that you might give up hope for the miracle you expected. Though not necessarily permissible in a friendship, I thought doing so would be both beneficial and constructive, and I was hoping that keeping it to myself would be for the good of others.

> The LORD is my rock, my fortress and my deliverer; my God is my rock, in whom I take refuge. He is my shield and the horn of my salvation, my stronghold.
>
> (Psalm 18:2 NIV)

The fact that, up to this point, I had withheld information about Wes's prognosis didn't seem to be a factor in whether our friends loved Wes or us. Claire had her own confession. She had surmised from my mood upon return from the doctor's office that day that I had received some dire news. Regardless of that perceived news, she continued to hold hope for Wes's complete recovery, never letting on that she knew. She, too, had silently shared my journey of despair.

The response to my confession was again an outpouring of compassion from those that we love. It was a testament to God's grace and analogous to His unyielding forgiveness for our transgressions.

I am now more convinced that the benefit is more apparent for the confessor than the one receiving it. It was good to know that now someone, everyone else, knew what I'd been solely privileged to for more than half a year.

23

Stuff

With that burden relieved, it was still necessary to continue finishing up the loose
ends created by Wes's passing. Each item had to be
remembered, recognized, reduced to a to-do list,
done, and marked off. I had wished that there had
been someone to whom I could have delegated the
exercise because some actions were more emotionally painful than others.

Still, with any death, there is business associated with it and that business must be done. I felt it
important that, if God was using us to communicate
to others the steps involved with losing a loved one,
then it was incumbent upon me to communicate
these issues.

By three methods we may learn wisdom:
First, by reflection, which is noblest;
second, by imitation, which is easiest; and
third, by experience, which is the bitterest.
—Confucius

The next week was difficult. "Stuff" had to be done. Wes's name had to be deleted off our gate list in the neighborhood. Wes had to be deleted off the insurance policies, auto and health. We filed for probate to close his accounts and received the authorization fairly quickly.

Doing those things caused me to recognize a certain anger about the necessity of it. I wasn't mad at Wes. I wasn't mad at God. I realized that I wasn't God. He, alone, was in charge of life and death. I was just mad at life in general, at how unfair it seems at times.

I still needed to cancel Wes's cell phone. I hadn't yet been able to do it. You see, if I called the number, I could still hear his voice on the voice mail. I'd not had the courage to do that. But I might find it at some point. And, once I did, I might want to do it often, for a long time. I wasn't ready for that yet. It was a link to him that I wasn't ready to relinquish just yet.

It was all very selfish on my part, the not letting go. We had been so blessed. God had been so good to us. Just think about it.

I had been able to retire a few years ago. Had I not, I wouldn't have been able to spend the past year with Wes. It was a difficult and trying time, but it was, in its own way, a special time. We — Wes, Claire, and I — communicated every day. When, late in his treatment, he had difficulty getting up by himself, I would stand over him and have him put his hands around my neck. We would stand together and, while his legs adjusted to the new position, I would just hold him and he me. Often we would just moan and tell each other how much we loved each other. All the jobs and fame in the world could not supplant the joy and comfort I received from those few moments. Wes was just like that, always wanting to express his love for the other person. What a blessing God gave us both in those few precious moments. I am truly blessed.

Sometimes, it seemed overwhelming, and Claire and I just wanted to get out of town. Maybe go to our place in Ponte Vedra. But there was so much to do; we didn't want to leave and then have to come back to more to do in the future. It was best if we did what had to be done first, and then, somehow, tried to relax at a future time. We persevered.

As I sat there one night and tried to reflect on God and His majesty, struggling to see the computer keyboard, the screen, or just life through my tears, I continued to recognize how good God is. How lucky was I to have a son like Wes? How lucky are we to have two other children whom we love dearly? How lucky are we to have friends who love us unconditionally and pray for us? How lucky were we to have good insurance that took care of the financial aspects of his illness so that it was not a worry? How lucky were we that we had a year of intimacy with Wes, regardless of the circumstances? How lucky are we that he is waiting for us and that we will see him again? How lucky are we that God grants us these things by grace and not by what we deserve? How lucky can we be?

It is by God's Word, promise, and hopefully His will that we attack each day. He gives us the wisdom to do those things that are necessary to face this life, however bitter it may be.

In him we were also chosen, having been predestined according to the plan of him

who works out everything in conformity
with the purpose of his will, in order that we,
who were the first to hope in Christ, might
be for the praise of his glory. And you also
were included in Christ when you heard the
word of truth, the gospel of your salvation.
Having believed, you were marked in him
with a seal, the promised Holy Spirit, who
is a deposit guaranteeing our inheritance
until the redemption of those who are God's
possession—to the praise of his glory. For
this reason, ever since I heard about your
faith in the Lord Jesus and your love for all
the saints, I have not stopped giving thanks
for you, remembering you in my prayers. I
keep asking that the God of our Lord Jesus
Christ, the glorious Father, may give you the
Spirit of wisdom and revelation, so that you
may know him better.

(Ephesians 1:11–17 NIV)

God revealed Himself to us in the blessings He
provided. Wes was marked with His seal, and we
are guaranteed an inheritance of redemption. How
lucky are we?

We continue to thank God for His blessings and pray that He will bless others as He has us. May He continue to grant all of us His wisdom, whether by reflection, imitation, or experience, because ours alone is insufficient.

No loss of a loved one is easy. Nor is the debilitating grief permanent. With that statement made, one would wonder, "When does the grief go away?" I don't think it ever does. The debilitating grief does seem to slip away in the middle of the night and go into hiding. It hides in a closet, a drawer, a song, or, in this case, for us, on a table in the basement or, for someone else, across a desk at the bank.

> He withdrew about a stone's throw beyond them, knelt down and prayed, "Father, if you are willing, take this cup from me; yet not my will, but yours be done."
>
> (Luke 22:41–42 NIV)

How many times did I voice that same type of prayer during Wes's illness? I continued to do so regarding the obligations of settling up Wes's affairs. Obviously, it was not God's will that the cup be taken from us and that's okay. What was difficult was knowing what God's will was regarding how we handled and dealt with the collateral.

Grief is a strange thing. When you think you have it under control, something you least expect conjures up the emotion. It might be a sight, a smell, a sound. That morning, it was the sound of a ping-pong ball hitting the floor. I was in an unfinished part of the house where I keep old records, searching for a written bank policy from years ago to take to a meeting. As I took one of the heavy books from the rack and plopped it on the table, it created a vibration that caused a ping-pong ball to roll off the table and bounce on the floor. I almost joined it there. You see, Wes was a terrific ping-pong player. He beat everybody, repeatedly. Recognizing that I'd no longer be able to hear him good-heartedly gloat over pounding someone into submission at the ping-pong table brought tears to my eyes. You just never know what will set you off. That did me.

God's will is so difficult to discern. I struggled with how I could come to know it. How was His will revealed?

Romans 8 offers some insight.

If we hope for what we do not yet have, we
wait for it patiently. In the same way, the
Spirit helps us in our weakness. We do not
know what we ought to pray for, but the
Spirit himself intercedes for us with groans
that words cannot express. And he who
searches our hearts knows the mind of the
Spirit, because the Spirit intercedes for the
saints in accordance with God's will.

(Romans 8:25–27 NIV)

I am results oriented and want results *now*!
Being patient was not and continues not to be my
strong suit. However, since I have no control and
have surrendered control, being patient is my only
option. Let me give you an example.

As I mentioned earlier, we received the order
from probate court allowing us to close Wes's
accounts, so the next Monday, I told Claire we had
to go close Wes's checking account. Reluctantly,
after a couple of deep breaths, we entered the bank
and sat down at the desk of the customer service
representative (CSR). She is someone with whom

I've dealt in the past. Prepared with copies of the order from the probate court and the death certificate, I handed her the checkbook and asked to close the account. She started dispatching my request without asking for any of the supporting documentation. It was only then I realized that with my name on the account as well she had no need for the support I had brought with me. Then, when I asked to close the credit card account, she called the 800 number and was asked by the person who answered to speak to me. After verifying some information, the woman on the phone attempted to confirm that I wanted to block the account. When I told her, "No, I want to close it," she inquired as to my reason. "Actually," I replied, "it was my son's account, and he is deceased." Hearing this, the CSR immediately teared up. I concluded my conversation with the credit card lady, accepting her sincerest condolences and the assurance that the account would be closed immediately, and the CSR, through her tears, said, "I am soooo sorry. Forgive me if I get emotional, but I lost my three daughters on Valentines' Day three years ago."

You see, I could ask, "Why me?" and feel sorry for myself, watching the world go on around me oblivious to my pain, not realizing that, in time, *if I am patient,* God will reveal others who did and are experiencing three times the pain that I feel. Crying with us, the CSR said, "They tell you that time eases the pain. That's a lie." I don't tell you this to minimize the loss of our son, but to put it in perspective. I hurt deeply for Wes's passing, but I hurt for this poor woman who lost her daughters as well. As hard as it was to grasp the void in our life, I can't begin to imagine the pain that manifested itself on her at that time and even today.

When I went back in the bank two days later, she immediately started messing with me, giving me a hard time, cementing a bond formed between us through our collective grief. I guess that explains Ecclesiastes 4.

> Two are better than one, because they have a good return for their work: If one falls down, his friend can help him up. But pity the man who falls and has no one to help him up!
> (Ecclesiastes 4:9–10 NIV)

Two are better than one. Four are better than two. One hundred are better than fifty.

As we meet others who have lost children, we find that the instant that common ground is discovered, you feel a bond. It's a weird bond, one that you don't want to have but one that you can't deny or resist. It's like belonging to a club that you've been forced to join. Simply recognizing a member breaks down any barrier between your hearts. It is only those who have been there who can truly empathize and share the devastation and the void created. The fortunate and uninitiated may say they understand, but their attempt at compassion falls on our ears as smoke.

I even had a woman say, "I've never lost a child, but I know how you feel. My dog died last month, and it was like losing a member of my family. It's so hard, isn't it?" I simply replied, "Yes, if you only knew."

What I really wanted to say was, "Lady, look. I've lost goldfish, hamsters, a dog, a dad, a brother, an infant daughter, and an adult son. No loss is fun, but until you've lost your own child, you haven't got a clue what heartache really is."

Fortunately, I thought better of it. In her defense it seems obvious that in her own discomfort at responding to our loss, she just didn't know what to say. As inappropriate as her comment had been, she was nonetheless attempting to reach out to us. For her to take the time to do so was appreciated.

Just as you think you're getting over the grief, however, it grabs you again. Grief has been likened to standing in the ocean, calf-deep with your back to the water. The gentle ebb and flow of the tide laps against your skin and gives you comfort and a false sense of peace. Then, when you least expect it, quietly and with little warning, a big wave rises up, catches you square in the back, and knocks you flat on your face. Caught in the swirl of the receding tide, it's difficult to stand up again, to gain your footing and to breathe again. But when you've regained your balance, you can once again assume the same position. This time, however, you know the wave of grief can and will come, but it won't be quite as big a surprise. It'll still knock you down, but you know that in time, with difficulty, you can stand again.

A wave caught Claire shortly after losing Wes while visiting a friend to look at wedding pictures. Initially, it was okay. Then it dawned on her that no wedding picture would ever include Wes. A big wave.

I dodged a wave when my dear friend Charles
Williams offered to lift Wes's voice mail from his
cell phone and e-mail it to me. He did so, and I was
able to save it without having to listen to it. Only
then, knowing I had it saved, could I cancel his cell
phone service.

Sean shared with me how the waves had
affected him. I asked if this situation had shaken or
strengthened his faith. Not surprisingly, his answer
was profound.

"My faith hasn't been shaken, but though my
faith didn't need a workout, it has been exercised.
I've always had the faith in my head and that's okay
when somebody else's friend or relative dies, but
when your own flesh and blood dies, you find your
faith can't be drawn upon in installments like it is
with others, but rather must be full time and not just
exercised but demonstrated."

Like the ocean, waves of grief have ripples that
affect others.

Claire and I have been blessed that Wes's
friends still keep us in their loop. One of Wes's best
friends was by the house within about a month of
the funeral, and as was our nature, we asked how
he was doing with it. He, too, had been dealing

with waves of grief. He, as is customary, wondered, "Why?" It's difficult for many to make sense from God's Word in Deuteronomy 29.

> The secret things belong to the LORD our God.
>
> (Deuteronomy 29:29)

The answer to the question "Why?" is one of those "secret things." He went on to describe where he was with it all. "Somewhere between overwhelmed with grief and wanting to join him."

Isn't that really where we all should want to be? Shouldn't we all want to be with Wes in heaven? Not today, but whenever God's secret things about our lives come to pass.

I can conjure up a wave and sometimes do, unintentionally, by thinking of the song played at Wes's celebration, "I Can Only Imagine."

Paraphrasing, in it the singer asks, "When I am in your presence, how will I react? Will I dance for you Jesus? Will I not be able to speak at all?"

I picture Wes and what he did when he met Jesus. Was he able to speak at all? Knowing Wes, he could and did. He embraced Jesus and said, as he did to all of us so many times, "I love you so much." But then, it might have been the other way around.

Claire mentioned on our walk one morning, as we surveyed the overcast day we were experiencing, "I like days like this. On sunny days, you're supposed to be up and happy, but on days like this it's okay to be where you are."

We recognize that it *is* okay to be where we are. We just stand in the ocean with our backs to the water, waiting for another wave.

Some days seem like we just trudge along in the mud, not making any real progress, wondering about the meaning of life. There was meaning before all this happened. There has got to be more than just getting through another day. We can hope. But for now, going through those daily motions may have to be enough.

At the time I wrote this, it had been six weeks.

The pain felt fresher than six weeks. I felt like I'd missed him for much, much longer. Claire had remarked at dinner a few nights earlier, "Wow. For about five minutes I felt normal." My question was, "And you felt guilty didn't you?"

She did. It comes and goes with the territory. But normalcy comes in installments right now. Just little snippets of feeling okay interspersed with the rain of feeling out of place in another world masquerading as the one in which we once lived. I don't know in which world we'll land, but whichever one it is, once it quits spinning, we'll have to stake claim to it. We'll adjust—eventually—sometime later.

At the cemetery, one of the pall bearers was approached by a nicely dressed gentleman in a suit who said, "You appear to be close to the Smiths. Would you see that they get this?" He then handed him a folder with Savannah College of Art & Design printed on the front. Inside was a business card identifying himself as the Dean of the School of Architecture at SCAD and a charcoal project Wes had done for one of his classes entitled "Light Reflections." Like the Lone Ranger, with a polite "thank you," the man disappeared. The picture was amazingly complex but delicately done, showing light reflections on a glass-paned window with the shadows of nearby trees playing off the window and the building. Obviously, the instructor found it to be important or he'd not have made a point to see that we had it. We are grateful for the professor's kindness. We've had it framed and hung by our bed along with a very kind letter from Paula Wallace, president of the school. We awake to Wes's "Light Reflections" each morning. And that's as it should be. We saw Wes's light reflected in so many places, in so many people, in so many circumstances, that it was hard to imagine that it had only been six weeks.

Experiencing a loss is felt by many to resemble a season. At the time, it is felt that it will pass. As it says in Ecclesiastes, "A time to be born, a time to die."

If it occurs like it does with my dad's passing (some twenty-two years ago), I just want to pick up the phone and call him. Realizing I can't, the question crosses my mind, "Is he still dead?" It just doesn't seem possible that someone to whom you are so extremely close and whom you love so deeply can go away for that long without returning. But then, we have to remember what David said in 2 Samuel when his son died, "I cannot bring him back but I can go to him." We just have to be patient and recognize that we can do that later.

Another friend of Wes's later confessed that she'd fallen victim to his voice mail once. I'd not succumbed to the urge to listen. I know what it says.

In his "I'm tough" rather monotone voice, he says, "Hey guys. I can't come to the phone. Leave me a message. I'll call you back—later."

No "good-bye, thanks for calling," just, "Later."

I suppose it's short for "See ya later." Nonetheless, it's simply put . . . "Later."

It's reminiscent of what Jesus said in John:

> Simon Peter asked him, "Lord, where are you going?" Jesus replied, "Where I am going, you cannot follow now, but you will follow later."
>
> (John 13:36 NIV)

I'm convinced that upon Wes's departure from this world, he had every intention of seeing us later. As Ernie Forrester, Wes's youth minister, said in the ceremony, Wes was most concerned that some of his friends wouldn't see him later, and Wes wanted to do his part to see that they would. He did his best in that regard.

For now, we have to be comfortable with the fact that where Wes went, we can't follow now. But we'll follow later.

Whether it's six weeks, six months, six years, or sixty years, we'll just lean on our faith and our friends (if they'll let us) to reflect on the light Wes left for us all to ponder.

At the end of week six, we went to Savannah. It took all we had to do some of the things we had to do. Cleaning out Wes's apartment in Savannah was one of those things.

Claire wanted to sort. There'd be time for that later. What we needed to do was to get it all, load it in the car, and get it home. We could sort later.

On the way to Savannah from Jacksonville, our radio was losing reception, so I started spinning the dial to find something to take our minds off what we were preparing to do. At some point, I picked up a station with a sermon by someone I didn't know and don't know to this day. However, his story seemed to have some relevance to our situation. It went something like this.

There was an island where all the feelings lived: Richness, Love, Happiness, Vanity, Sadness, and Knowledge. There was news that the island was going to sink and that all the feelings had to find a way off the island.

All departed except Love who loved the
island and wanted to stay and try to save the
beautiful island. When it became apparent
that the island was, in fact, sinking, Love
tried to find a way off. First, Richness came
sailing by in a big, expensive boat. But
when Love asked if he could ride, Richness
declined stating that there was too much
gold and silver on board to provide room
for Love. Next, Vanity came sailing by in a
glorious vessel but said Love was already
wet and just wouldn't fit in. Happiness
sailed by next but was too joyous in celebration to even hear Love's cry. Sadness then
was asked by Love but replied, "No, I just
need to be alone." Just as Love was about
to give up, an elder came by and offered
Love a ride. So happy to have a way off the
sinking island, Love failed to even ask the
name of the elder who provided relief. The
elder safely deposited Love on dry land and
disappeared. Later, once safe, Love wanted
to thank the elder for his kindness. So Love
asked Knowledge who had been so kind.
Knowledge replied to Love that the elder

was in fact Time. "Why?" Love questioned, "would Time save me when none of the others would?" Knowledge answered, "Only Time can reveal how great Love is."

Time does, in fact, allow love for others to deepen. Many would think that the year we spent with Wes as we tried to find a cure for his illness would have been intolerable. To the contrary, the time we spent allowed our love for him to grow. Now, in his absence, we recognized how much we loved him and continued to love him. It seemed to exacerbate the grief.

We are prepared to grieve for a long time, because only that time will reveal how great our love is.

Our love for Wes will endure the passage of time. That's as it should be, just as Jesus' love for us endures. Through Him, we can conquer our grief and all the things of this earth.

In all these things we are more than conquerors through him who loved us. For I am convinced that neither death, nor life, nor angels, nor rulers, nor things present, nor things to come, nor powers, nor height, nor depth, nor anything else in all creation, will be able to separate us from the love of God in Christ Jesus our Lord.

(Romans 8:37–39)

24

Coping and a Trophy

The e-mail updates had been presented in regular installments for a little over two years. From the first one, I feared I would be intruding on other people's generally happy lives. It was not my intention to place periodic blemishes on their otherwise tranquil existence. Repeatedly, I asked that they tell me if the e-mails were the intrusions I feared. No one ever said to stop. On numerous occasions, I was encouraged to continue sending them and send them more often as they mentioned how the updates provided them with a reality check of what was truly important in life. Life was more than just making the carpool and dealing with everyday struggles. It was, at times, life and death. Likewise, they felt that the series might be of some help to others who encountered similar trials. Nonetheless, grief was taking its toll on my ability to write as frequently and provide anything helpful, so I decided to throttle back the e-mails. Here's how that was conveyed. Once again, God placed us at the right place at the right time to receive a story that was pertinent to what we wanted to express.

> On the day I called, you answered me, you increased my strength of soul.
>
> (Psalm 138:3)

It had been almost a year and two months since we first called out to our friends when Wes was diagnosed. Without hesitation, they stepped in and made our lives large with their strength and God's strength. How great was their love. We would be forever grateful.

As weeks went by, we, or more specifically I, called out again and again. They continued to step in with strength, support, and prayers to provide us the support we needed to face the next week. They continually showed us God's love.

I wrote the updates, giving hope, asking for hope for ourselves, and attempting to help all to understand the terror and comfort we felt with each passing week. We collectively prayed for miracles, miracles that we thought valid. But more often than not, miracles we sought were to keep our son on this side of heaven rather than to let him go home. We were uncomfortable with the "going home" aspect of it all. To some degree, we still are.

I had heard a story by a TV pastor while we were in Ponte Vedra.

In late summer, there was a young mother who was diagnosed with a terminal illness and given only six months to live. She had an eight-year-old son and didn't know how to tell him. One day, the preacher came by, and she asked if he would tell her son and he agreed.

"Jimmy," the pastor said, "your momma is going away. She's going to be with Jesus."

"When?" asked Jimmy.

"In a while," said the pastor, "when all the leaves on the trees are gone."

Jimmy seemed to take the news rather stoically.

When the pastor came back in late December to call on the ailing mother, he inquired about Jimmy and how he was doing.

"I don't really know," said the mother. "I don't see him very much. He's out in the backyard."

The pastor exited the back door, looked around, and, to his amazement, didn't see Jimmy.

He called out, "Jimmy!"

"Up here!" came a cry.

The pastor asked, "Jimmy, what are you doing up in that tree?"

"Pastor, I'm just tying on some more leaves."

I think we tied until our fingers bled for Wes. But isn't that what Christ did for us? It seems easier to reconcile when I realize that, despite how much I loved Wes, God loves *him* more. Despite how much Wes loves us, God loves *us* more. When in a skirmish over who loves who more, God is *going* to win. Hands down. Every time. I have to accept that.

> [Love] bears all things, believes all things,
> hopes all things, endures all things. Love
> never ends.
>
> (1 Corinthians 13:7–8)

How true that is. Our love for Wes, our love for others, and our collective love for our Lord and Savior Jesus Christ does not end.

But other things do, like the e-mail updates. I wanted them to be relevant and uplifting and hopeful and to connect the readers with God in some fashion each week. As we continued to travel down the grief path, I was finding it less reasonable to reach those expectations.

Earlier, I received an e-mail from Scotty, the young man who so eloquently sang "I Can Only Imagine" at Wes's celebration. It included a song track. The song was written by Wes, put to music by Scotty, and accompanied on violin by one of Wes's best friends, Brandon. The title is "'Til the End," and it speaks of love until the end. How appropriate.

How relevant. I owe a debt to these friends of Wes's 'til the end. What a great way to honor their friend.

'Til the End

Can you tell me
What's happening
It's never felt this true
Until I met you
You make me laugh, you set me free,
You complete every part of me.
From the first time you held my hand,
I knew I would love you 'til the end.
Not a day goes by
That you don't run through my mind,
And when I hold you near,
I'll tell you I'll always be right here.
Even through the heartache and pain
Even when the heavens rain,
Now, separated,
Well, I still waited.
The feelings I still have for you
Will never fade away
Neither will the love so true that
Now I'm strong enough to say

I knew this "first" would come and when. It was one of those "firsts" that was preordained from the day Wes died. It was simply unavoidable.

I've heard it said and believe it to be true that "coincidence occurs when God chooses to no longer remain anonymous."

Claire sees coincident symbols in things that I sometimes don't recognize. She and I have a first-floor condo in Ponte Vedra Beach, Florida, that we bought in January of 2002. It's on the south end of the building and faces both the ocean and the complex next door. When the developers were tying the two complexes together by way of common landscaping at the bottom of the little knoll between our complex and the next, the developer placed three palm trees in a grouping, each taller than the next. It made for a nice view to see the trees, then the dunes, then the beach, and then the ocean. Oddly enough, the smallest tree had been abused by the grass cutters as they would come down the hill and allow the lawnmower to graze against the trunk, knocking a little piece of bark away each time until the base of the smallest tree had a diameter of about six inches supporting a trunk of twelve or so inches. Then last July, when the two hurricanes came through, the winds apparently were more than the little tree could stand and it broke and lay on the ground next to the other two. When Claire and I went down in March to decompress and arrange to clean out Wes's apartment in Savannah, the little tree was gone. The last time we visited, Claire confided in me how she had always known that this was the right condo for us because the three palm trees represented our three children. The smallest tree was less healthy and coincidentally so was Wes. Coincident with the hurricanes of 2004, Wes relapsed and the smallest tree fell down. In February, they took the little tree away. Coincidence? I choose to think not.

August 1, 2005, would have been Wes's twenty-third birthday. August 2 marked six months since his death. Wes lived 8,213 days. That's twenty-two and a half years. Not *nearly* twenty-two and a half years, not *about* twenty-two and a half years, but *exactly* twenty-two and a half years. Coincidence? Maybe. Maybe not.

Claire and I have dealt with this in the best way we know how. We sometimes have to beg out of invitations just because we need to reflect and don't feel like being light and jovial. We've changed our pace. We both have occasional bad days for different reasons, but coincidentally, we both have our bad days on the same days. At times we feel that we should be over it because the weight of missing Wes is so heavy on our hearts and minds that surely we should feel a reprieve. Not so.

Claire and I went to Ponte Vedra in June just to clear our heads and attempt to establish some normalcy. To our dismay, Grief followed us down there in a truck and brought his whole family, Depression, Sorrow, Anger, and Despair. For different reasons we were both emotionally trashed from Friday through Tuesday. Awaking Wednesday morning and feeling overwhelmed by the same feelings as on the previous days, I checked my computer for e-mails and had a message from my friend whose wife had died the day before Wes. As an attachment to his e-mail was a copy of the sermon his preacher had delivered the previous Sunday dealing with grief.

> Love comes with a cost. Its penalty is grief. The depth of your grief is a direct reflection of the depth of your love for the one you lost. The more you love them, the

more deeply and longer you will grieve
when you lose them.

You can't be done with grief until grief
is done with you.

That very minute, those thoughts took purchase
in my heart and gave me permission to be "not
okay." It wasn't up to me to get over it. When grief
gets done with me, if it does, I'll know it.

Almost giddy, I called for Claire and had her
come in and read the sermon. She had the same
reaction. Things have been improving since then
simply because we know it's okay to not be okay.
Was it a coincidence that my friend sent that e-mail
to us on that day? I choose to think not.

Lastly, throughout Wes's illness and passing, the
love and prayers and concern shown by others lifted
us up and provided us the strength to face each
day. Since his death, that continued support was
so needed and welcome, we wanted to thank those
folks for it. Wes's friends rallied around us and
accepted us, Claire and I, as their friends, coming
for visits, calling on Father's Day, Mother's Day,
today, any day, sending cards, bringing flowers,
offering hugs and encouragement, and allowing us

to lean on each other as we collectively tried to get through it. It seemed apparent that the people who make a difference in your life are not the ones with the most credentials, the most money, or the most awards. They are the ones who care.

Those of us who try to control things need to recognize that God, not us, is in complete control and our fretting over every issue is neither justified nor productive. Snoopy's creator sums it up pretty succinctly.

> Don't worry about the world coming to
> an end today. It's already tomorrow in
> Australia. —Charles Schultz

As I struggled with my own control issues, that comment was e-mailed to me. Coincidence? I think not.

In the middle of September, we reached a milestone for which Wes and we had been working for more than two years.

As I've indicated so many times before, we learned during Claire's bout with breast cancer and during Wes's fight with leukemia that cancer patients live their lives in installments. The completion of each round of chemo grants you a reprieve until the next test or doctor's appointment. Then you wait for results. Once you get the all clear, you can breathe fairly normally until the next appointment nears. The installment is due.

During the illness, hope comes in installments as well. It fills in between the installments of worry. It's a roller-coaster ride of highs being made of hope and lows being made of fear. You do, indeed, live your life in installments.

Grief is like that too. I've come to realize that you grieve in installments. But unlike your house payment, car note, or utility bill, grief installments are irregular. Initially, they are frequent. As frequent as every breath you take. Grief seems to sit on your chest and prevents you from taking in any air. After some time of exercising your lung muscles, struggling to breathe, grief moves off your chest and just occasionally, with varying frequency, smacks you in the heart hard enough to take your breath away and possibly take you to your knees. One of those installments was due. I'm pretty convinced that this mortgage that grief has on our hearts will never be paid up. We'll continue making installments until we join Wes.

But, then, closure comes in installments too. We experienced an episode that week that validated that point.

Wes was personified by his car, a 2002 Honda S2000 convertible that was white with a red interior. He loved that car. He and his friends worked on that car often with superior results in an effort to make it a show car. Wes did the same with his previous car and was successful in winning a trophy at NOPI Nationals. All through Wes's illness and treatments, he had focused on getting his car ready for the NOPI Nationals held in September each year. As I mentioned, while Wes was lying in his bed at Emory and receiving chemotherapy, he would call out customized parts to his friends or me so that we could make a list on the marker board in his room. He knew what they would cost, how they were to be installed, and timed everything so that, upon his temporary release from the hospital, he could have the items installed. And then, if he was really persuasive, he might get a "pass" the weekend of NOPI, take his car down, and get the coveted trophy. The previous year, about the same time, the Thursday before he was to attend NOPI on Friday, having installed all the equipment as promised, another driver turned into him on Satellite Boulevard and caused significant damage to Wes's car, rendering it unshowable at NOPI. His dream that he had held on to for so long and fought for so hard wasn't going to happen.

But it did. It wasn't easy, but it did. Wes didn't get his car out of the shop until December. Then he took it to get it turbocharged. He never got to drive it again. That shop kept it until after Wes had passed away. We took the car to a motorsports shop to finish it up. They did a great job. However, there were some telltale signs of the previous repair guys that came back to haunt us. One day while I was driving it, the turbo came loose, sucked the gasket up into it, and ruined a rather expensive turbo. The shop quickly and efficiently fixed that. Then, about three weeks later while riding in the rain southbound on I-85 in five o'clock traffic at an uncharacteristic fifty-eight miles per hour with an eighteen-wheeler on my bumper in the left-hand lane, the car hydroplaned, spun twice, missed the guardrail by about six inches, and slid backward off the right side of the road into a ditch and nestled gently up against a treelined knoll. The only casualties of the accident were the fiberglass side skirts

Wes had added to the car. Undeterred, I found
the vendor for the side skirts, got them, and had
one of Wes's friends to paint and install them on
Wednesday of the next week. On Friday the motorsports folks took the car to the NOPI Nationals
competition in Hampton, Georgia, on Wes's behalf,
and in his memory, represented the car and won a
trophy *and* oversaw the car receiving a designa-
tion of being an NOPI Elite automobile, a designa-
tion that follows the car for the rest of its life and
provides special privileges for the car and its owner
at every NOPI-sponsored show in the nation. I
know Wes was smiling.

Claire and I were too. That event represented a
huge installment in the closure of what Wes wanted
done. We were relieved.

It was a thrill to finally accomplish what Wes
had tried so desperately to achieve. Even to receive
the award posthumously held a degree of gratifica-
tion steeped in sorrow for his absence. However,
with that task now completed, we were able to put
some closure on the ownership of his Honda S2000.
Now it could be sold, and it was, to Wes's dear
friend Ryan who loves the car as Wes did. For that
we are thankful.

While leaving a bank in Buford later the next week, two lanes to my right was a white Pontiac convertible with a black top. To my surprise, on a decal covering almost the entire rear window, I read, "What is your greatest fear? Wes Smith, August 1, 1982–February 2, 2005." It took my breath away. I didn't know who it was and wasn't in a position to catch them. After asking around for a few days, one of Wes's friends identified the owner for us. Why the question? At Wes's ceremony, Ernie Forrester, our minister of youth, described a conversation with Wes while he was in the hospital. "What's your greatest fear, Wes?" To which Wes replied, "That some of my friends won't be in heaven with me."

So we do, indeed, live our lives in installments. It is important for us to realize that this life on this earth is just an installment. It is just the dash between 1982 and February on that decal. The impressions we make with our "dash" may change someone else's life or more. I hope I can make a difference with my dash; I know Wes did with his.

25

The Last "Firsts"
and the Last "Last"

As our first Thanksgiving rolled around after Wes's passing, honestly, we were ambivalent about how thankful we could be considering the fact that we'd have an empty chair at the dining room table. With that anticipation and reflection on the things we indeed knew we were thankful for, I tried to focus on my gratefulness.

Of course, we were thankful for our children and the manner in which they had rallied around us that first year.

We were thankful for our families and our extended families and the support they had provided during our loss.

We were thankful for Wes's friends who continued to visit and care for us, almost as if Wes were still here. For the little tributes they pay to him and us by showing up in one of Wes's shirts or jackets and proudly proclaiming its origin. We were thankful that they still felt comfortable to come over unannounced, raid our refrigerator or cookie jar, or stay for dinner. We were thankful when they wanted to just hang out alone in Wes's room.

We were thankful that Wes's car went to the NOPI car show and came back with a trophy. We were thankful that one of his dearest friends bought Wes's car and now pampers it as Wes did. We were proud that he observes Wes's 36-degree rule. (If it's 36 degrees or warmer, the top is down!)

We were thankful for the yet unmet female friend who had emblazoned on the rear window of her convertible, "What is your greatest fear? Wes Smith, August 1, 1982–February 2, 2005." And we were thankful for the testimony those words provided.

We were thankful for the twenty-two and a half years we had with Wes. They were all wonderful. Most of all, we were thankful for having had that last year with him, to love him and to have him

love us. I can't imagine how difficult a sudden
and tragic loss of a child must be. Neither feels
tolerable.

We were thankful for God's words and the
comfort that they provided when we struggled to
find words or meaning for ourselves. And how,
when we found ourselves at a complete and total
loss, somehow, someway, God made those words
known to us, with no effort from ourselves, by
having them show up in a card, letter, e-mail, radio
announcement, or TV show. It was at times like
those that we could see how real, loving, omni-
scient, and omnipresent our God truly is.

We continued to be thankful for our friends
every day, not just on Thanksgiving. Their
continued love and support and words of encouragement had been the salve necessary to help us
heal. The wounds were still there and the scars
would remain forever, but through their compassionate ministry to us, we tried to heal appropri-
ately. We were continually overwhelmed at the
depth and breadth of their friendship and love for
us and often felt unworthy of such dedication. They
always seemed to know what we needed and when
we needed it, and they provided it so selflessly that

they instilled in us the courage and support that we needed to carry on.

We were thankful for countless blessings too numerous to mention: food, shelter, beautiful sunsets, flowers, and more. We have been, as God has promised, blessed beyond measure and mostly for the blessing of His Son and the sacrifice of His life for our sins. I can only imagine how God must have felt on that day, but then I recognize that Wes is with Him and His Son, and it's a place we can only hope to be one day. We were then, and remain today, thankful for God's plan, whatever that might be.

Despite our fear that it would not, the sun did come up on Thanksgiving morning. We were faced with how we would adapt to repairing the hole at our dining room table and the one in our hearts. It had occurred to us to call our dear friends Bob and Charlotte to see if they'd like to have Thanksgiving dinner with us. It just so happened that their children were celebrating with the in-laws this year, and they had no one with whom to share the day. They accepted our invitation.

As we sat down to eat and it was obviously time for me to pray, I didn't know how I was going to do it without getting terribly emotional, but God stepped in. I managed to thank God for those things for which we were grateful and for His help in bearing up during our losses and for His grace when we experienced gains. It seemed the appropriate thing to say and mean it.

And so we ate. More than we should have. There were no empty chairs at the table and more than a few empty plates when dessert and coffee came around. I was fearful as we pushed back from the table that the lull that is so customary after every Thanksgiving meal might lead to conversation about Wes. People tend to get philosophical when they have a full stomach. So, as we cleared off the table, I was anxious and somewhat afraid of what the rest of the day held for us.

About that time, the back door opened, and Ryan said, "Hellooooo!" And in he came. A few minutes later, more of Wes's friends came. And then more, until by late afternoon, we had a house full of kids: Ryan, Brandon, Patrick, Raivo, and more. They were laughing, cutting up, and telling stories about Wes (some we hadn't heard and some we probably wish we never had). Our house was alive.

Some left, went and got their girlfriends, and came back. They stayed, they ate, they drank, they were having a good time . . . with us. How kind. How thoughtful. How unexpected. How appreciated.

Finally, with a few stragglers still left, Claire and I turned to the remaining few and said, "We're going to bed. We love ya. We'll see you soon. Turn the lights off and lock up when you leave." And with a series of systematic hugs, we went to bed. Once there, we looked at each other, and I said, "I really didn't know what to expect this morning when we got up, and I was really scared about how this day would turn out. But, you know, it turned out okay. It was a good day. One better than I'd have ever imagined. God is good." With a smile and a kiss, we went to sleep.

The holiday season was then officially under way, and we went about our Christmas shopping and preparation with a little less anxiety now that we knew that we could, conceivably, get through a holiday without being puddles on the floor.

Every Christmas has its own significance. For the Smith family, last year's Christmas held a special place in our hearts. This first one following Wes's death would too.

This Christmas brought to mind another story about Wes. Even now, when I think about it, I find it hard to believe. I don't truly think I would believe it, had it not happened to me.

During the summer of 2003 (I think), Wes and a friend had come to me one evening as I was sitting on the front porch having a cigar. Wes's friend was in some financial distress, and Wes asked for my help. "How much do you need?" I asked and was told that $900 would handle the immediate difficulty.

I excused myself and went and got $1,500, handed it to the young man, and said, "Here's what you need, plus a little more. Pay me back when you can." He and Wes were both appreciative.

During the next year or so, I would inquire of Wes about his friend. No conversation was ever engaged about the money, but Wes knew why I inquired. No offer of repayment came.

After Wes was diagnosed and during the summer of 2004, during one of Wes's releases from the hospital when once again I was sitting outside having a cigar, Wes came to me alone and handed me $1,500 in cash.

"I got your money," he said.

"How did that happen?" I asked.

"I just went over to his house and got it from him," Wes answered.

My response caught Wes off guard.

"Wes," I said, "I can't take the money from you. Don't misunderstand; I appreciate your efforts on my behalf, but he needs to hand me the money personally, just as it was given to him."

After some discussion, Wes dejectedly relented and went on about his business. Nothing was ever said again about the money by Wes or his friend.

The night of Wes's funeral, lots of folks came back to the house. Among them was Wes's friend. Overwrought with the loss of his best friend, he approached Claire who very candidly said, "You need to find Smitty and apologize." The friend found me downstairs that night and approached me with tears in his eyes and said, simply, "I'm sorry." I sat on a stool in the den downstairs, and he sat on the floor in front of me, and I offered the explanation I thought he wanted.

"Look," I said, "I want you to understand why I couldn't accept the money from Wes that you'd given him. You see, I never intended to take that money back from you. The impression that it was a 'loan' was merely a test. I wanted to find out if you'd offer it back to me; it was a test of integrity, so to speak. Because of that, it needed to be done personally so that I could tell you that I loved you and that it wasn't a loan, but a gift, and that you could keep it."

The friend looked at me with this dumbfounded expression and said, "What are you talking about?"

"What do you mean?" I asked.

He replied, "I never gave Wes any money to give you."

In that instant, Wes's friend and I both came to the same startling conclusion. Wes offered to pay the debt of his friend to receive forgiveness for the friend from his father.

Wow!

We both burst into tears.

Wes, anonymously and without provocation or expectation of anything in return, loved his friend so much that he was willing to pay his debts for him.

It seemed appropriate that we recognize that, during the holiday season, we celebrate the birth of Jesus Christ who came to do the same for us. Without provocation, without request, He came and gave His life to pay our debts. Wes had apparently learned that lesson well enough to try to exercise it in his life for his friend.

We've said for a long time that Wes was God's child. Claire and I can't take credit for this episode in Wes's life. It was Christ's presence in Wes that caused this to play out. God was in the details. Had I accepted the money from Wes that night, we might have never recognized the parallel created by Wes's actions.

It would be my prayer that everyone would think about the Christ in Christmas all year, not just at Christmas. I know it made me want to be more like Wes. I wanted to forgive somebody. I wanted to pay someone else's debt. Maybe, there is someone you need to forgive. The repayment of a debt over which you may have been laboring, that you recognize holds little true significance in the big picture, needs to be forgiven. Maybe it's just to make you think. I know it did me.

"For God so loved the world . . ." (John 3:16). His Son came so that our son has a place to wait for us. I had meant to relay that episode by e-mail to our friends many times over the months since Wes's passing, but, somehow, some way, every time I'd start to write it, there was another story begging to be told. I was never at a loss for what to write. God managed each week or month to place square in front of me an angel, an episode, a trial, or a miracle. Attached to each seemed to be a message that God wanted me to convey. Please don't misunderstand my words.

I'm no prophet. I'm no special writer. I almost failed English composition my freshman year in college. The professor handed back one of my papers with an inscription in red punctuated by an exclamation point that stated, "How did you ever get out of high school?!"

No, I'm just some guy whom God has apparently chosen to convey a few things about life. He has seemingly given me some clarity of vision whereby I am able to recognize His hand in the fabric of our lives and then, to my surprise, He expects, or more properly, compels me to write about it.

Trust me. I couldn't make this stuff up. Truth is often stranger than fiction. And so it was with the previous account. Had it not happened to me, I would not have believed it. It is retold as it happened. He and I have become very close.

I just wrote as God led me to do. Each time I sat before the keyboard to provide an account, God guided my hands and my thoughts and my words. But I knew that there would come a day when we would finally reach the last "first," and the storytelling would stop. That occurred on February 2, 2006. Destiny prevailed. Here's how.

That day marked the last "first" and marked the last "last.

February 2nd will always be Groundhog Day to most, the day our dog Sydney was born, and the day that Wes sang and danced for Jesus. I can only imagine how he reacted when they met, but if I know Wes, and I think I do, Wes would have done it all: he would have sung, danced, and worshipped.

So February 2nd marked the last "first" for us. Oh sure, there's probably a stray out there somewhere of which we aren't even aware that will sneak up on us, catch us on our blind side, and knock us to our emotional knees when we least expect it, but we've managed to get through the other "firsts" without too much scarring. Mother's Day and Father's Day were especially difficult as was Wes's birthday. We dreaded Thanksgiving, but Wes's friends came in all afternoon and evening and enveloped us in their love, laughter, and nonsense. We didn't know how much we needed them, but they helped us through a lot of tough times that year, and we grew to love them more than we had before (if that's possible). Due to loving family and friends, Christmas and New Year's Eve were as uneventful as you could imagine considering the void created where Wes had been. So we came to this—the last "first."

As I sat there leaking, as I often did when relaying our stories, I realized that I continued to do so, maybe not as much for the loss of our dear Wes, but because of the feeling of unworthiness for the continued outpouring of love, compassion, and affection of our friends and Wes's who had now become ours. Those friends had become the knot at the end of our emotional rope. They called, appeared, wrote, smiled, and hugged just when we needed encouragement. It had been never ending and ever needed.

So we took heart in a couple of things at that milestone.

One, we don't ask "Why?" as much anymore. We leave that up to God as it says in Deuteronomy 29:29, "The secret things belong to the LORD our God." We've become more comfortable with the understanding that "Why?" is just one of those "secret things" that is part of God's much larger plan for our life than we can grasp at this time. He will reveal that to us when we see Him as Wes has. We'll just have to live with that knowledge.

The other knowledge that God provides for times like these can be found in the books of Ecclesiastes and Nehemiah.

> For everything there is a season, and a time for every matter under heaven: a time to be born, and a time to die; a time to plant, and a time to pluck up what is planted; a time to kill, and a time to heal; a time to break down, and a time to build up; a time to weep, and a time to laugh; a time to mourn, and a time to dance.
>
> (Ecclesiastes 3:1–4)

> This day is sacred to our Lord. Do not grieve, for the joy of the Lord is your strength.
>
> (Nehemiah 8:10 NIV)

We try to go forward each day with the recognition that each day is sacred and all the strength that we will ever need can be found in our Lord and Savior.

Besides, I've heard it said that you can't really consider something or someone lost if you know where they are. We know where Wes is today, and where he will be for all our tomorrows. We will be with him again, and it's only our impatience that makes that wait so difficult.

And so if we can release our grief, we come to our last "last."

Shortly after Wes passed away, one of his dearest friends, Brandi Romine, approached us at church one Sunday and handed us an envelope. It had been a senior design graphics project at Auburn University for her to design a logo for a fictitious, nonprofit organization. Recognizing her affection for Wes and her understanding of what he had been through, Brandi devised the WES Foundation: When Everyone Survives. The logo is done in red, white, and gray (Wes's favorite colors) and depicts the struggle between red and white blood cells that accompanies the disease which is leukemia and the research that needs to be done to one day overcome the disease. Brandi's talent as a graphic artist and her creative spirit fueled ours and the When Everyone Survives Foundation has been created. It is a 501c3, tax-deductible charity dedicated to helping fund leukemia research. Sean has been serving as the Executive Director of the foundation and is uniquely qualified for that role as he studied premed extensively in college and can converse with equal ease with laypeople and professionals alike. Our website has been developed and is an initiative to serve as a one stop shop for leukemia patients, caregivers, family, friends, and loved ones. It can be found at wesfoundation.org or WhenEveryoneSurvives.org. Great strides have been made over the last thirty years with the treatment and cure rate of leukemia, and it is our fervent hope that we can, through the generosity of ourselves and others, play some part in the discovery that finds the day when everyone survives.

It is through this mission that we will attempt to complete the work God began in Wes. As it says in Philippians 1:6: "And I am convinced and sure of this very thing, that He who began a good work in you will continue until the day of Jesus Christ [right up to the time of His return], developing [that good work] and perfecting and bringing it to full completion in you" (AMP).

I don't know how anyone could get through this type of trauma without a strong faith in a higher power and the love of friends. Our friends rose to the challenge and prayed us through. In closing I offer a prayer for you. It's the same prayer we said for Wes as we left him that last night at the funeral home.

The LORD bless you and keep you;

the LORD make his face to shine upon you,
and be gracious to you;
the LORD lift up his countenance upon you,
and give you peace.
Amen.
(Numbers 6:24–26)

To sum this all up, triskaidekaphobia still causes my heart to take a jump when Friday the thirteenth draws near. But what we have come to realize is that the fear of Friday the thirteenth gave us one last year to spend with our son. Allow me to explain.

Claire's fear of having Wes travel on Friday the thirteenth caused her to insist that he come home on Thursday night. Had he waited until Friday, the doctor would have been closed by the time Wes arrived home (they close at 1:00 PM on Fridays). He didn't seem that ill, and we'd have probably decided to wait until Monday for him to see the doctor. During that time between Friday and Monday, his counts would have escalated far beyond the 140,000 that they were found to be on Friday afternoon to numbers approaching 250,000, and Wes would have likely been blind or dead by Monday the fifteenth.

I guess there is such a thing as healthy fear, and in this case it seemed to have provided a substantial benefit. There is also a thought that all fear is irrational. I would think that if you have read this account, you would agree that there are times when fear is very, very rational.

It is my prayer that no one should be required to go through what we did with Wes. However, if, God forbid, it should happen, we pray that you'll remember the analogy I heard. Jesus is there to "hold your coat." He knows of the pending fight, shows up by your side, and simply says, "Let Me hold your coat." As you fight, He's there to cheer you on, and when it's all done, He'll bandage you up and even carry you out. The fight itself is yours, necessary for reasons not yet known. He is with you from start to finish, but it's your fight. Despite how it looks in the midst of the battle, you'll come through stronger with His love, the love of your family, and the love and prayers of your friends.

Thank you for enduring this journey with us, whether it was up to the minute, by our side, or just reading the account after the fact. It did take endurance because the journey was arduous to read, to hear about, or to live. It's a journey I wish not to make again but know now that I can with friends and God by my side.

Epilogue

Throughout our journey we seemed to continually recognize that certain people had certain jobs to do in their lives. Betty Eadie, in her book *Embraced by the Light*, shared her recollection from "the other side."

> *I saw many spirits who would only come to the earth for a short time, living only hours, or days after their birth. They were as excited as the others, knowing that they had a purpose to fulfill. I understood that their deaths had been appointed before their births—as were all of ours. These spirits did not need the development that would result from longer mortality, and their deaths would provide challenges that would help*

*their parents grow. The grief that comes
here is intense but short. After we are united
again, all the pain is washed away, and only
the joy of our growth and togetherness is
felt.*

This seems to explain a lot about those jobs.
Megan's job was to prepare us for Wes's death. And
Wes's job was to get his parents, and more specifically his dad, out of the blocks toward doing something meaningful for others.

In an effort to continue Wes's work in his
absence, I embrace the verse in Philippians:

I am confident of this, that the one who
began a good work among you will bring it
to completion by the day of Jesus Christ.
(Philippians 1:6)

It is with that spirit that we have created the
**When Everyone Survives Foundation (or WES
Foundation).** The name and logo were the brain-
child of one of Wes's dearest friends as part of a
college graphics arts project. On a lark, she gave the
design to us, and we have made it a reality.

When Everyone Survives is a not-for-profit 501c(3) charity dedicated to finding a cure or cures for leukemia so that no other set of parents will be forced to endure the trauma and tragedy we did. Significant numbers of leukemia patients survive today where virtually none survived thirty-five years ago. If that rate of progress continues, statistically, a cure for all those stricken with the disease can't be far off. We intend to put all our efforts into finding that cure.

It is our plan that each year, as we decide how our funds can be distributed to leukemia researchers, our Medical Advisory Board, made up of leukemia researchers, oncologists, and physicians, will collectively choose where those funds will go so that they will be put to use in the most productive and efficient manner. You can find out more about the foundation, what we do, and why we do it by accessing our website www.wheneveryonesurvives.org.

All author's proceeds from the sale of this book are going to the When Everyone Survives Foundation. It is our fervent prayer that through those contributions, the continued fund-raising efforts of the foundation, and donations from folks like you we will soon find a day When Everyone Survives.

Acknowledgments

I would be remiss if I didn't thank a few people who have shepherded me through this process. Countless friends read the manuscript during the process and provided valuable input but two people have been instrumental in seeing that I had a work product worthy of reading.

First, upon the suggestion of a mutual friend, Calvin Edwards accepted the challenge of reviewing my work early on in the process. Through his valuable insight and persistent dedication, he had me complete several rewrites to take this work from a mere compilation of e-mails to a conversation with you about our journey. Words are inadequate to express my appreciation to him for his care, concern, and compassion. Thank you, Calvin, for the value of your experience and most of all for your friendship.

And, lastly, I'd like to thank Amy Clark, the editor, who took a novice writer's work and honed it into something presentable. There were countless edits that required her to suggest changes that made the work much better than I could have imagined without limiting "my voice" in the telling of the story. To do that takes immeasurable talent, and I will always be indebted to her for her efforts on my behalf.

I am a better man for having worked with these two extraordinary individuals and *Later* is far better for it.

"Later."

Breinigsville, PA USA
26 October 2009
226502BV00001B/2/P

9 781615 792689